Today homoeopathy is a frequently misunderstood branch of the art of medicine. Any misapprehensions that the interested doctor or layman may have are dispelled in Dr Blackie's lively and informative book.

`The homoeopathic doctor studies the whole person in all his or her aspects: the individual idiosyncrasies, reactions to heat and cold, the responsiveness to weather and food, sleep and work patterns, age and environment, are all taken into account. The homoeopathic doctor knows that the infection is there, but he knows further why it is reacting in that particular manner in that particular person. The homoeopathic doctor's prime concern is the patient, not the patient's symptoms.

For nearly two hundred years the concept that Like will cure Like has been tested over and over again. And repeatedly it has been proved right. From the beginning it was found in homoeopathic testing that no single symptom was sufficient to indicate the remedy for a total cure. It has been shown that by taking the mass of symptoms found in testing and matching the reactions between the healthy and the ill, that a true remedy for the entire individual organism can be prescribed. Today throughout the world many general practitioners as well as specialists are turning towards homoeopathy.

Dr Margery Blackie was appointed physician to the Queen in 1969. From 1965 she was the Dean of the Faculty of Homoeopathy, and in 1966 became Honorary Consulting Physician to the Royal London Homoeopathic Hospital. There is a tradition of medicine in her family; one of the most influential homoeopathic doctors in the last century was her uncle, Dr Crompton-Burnett. Dr Blackie retired in 1979.

By gracious permission of
Her Majesty The Queen,
I have been allowed to put the picture which was taken at a Homoeopathic Reception into the book. This reception was held at The Guildhall on 20th October 1970, when forty-three homoeopathic doctors were presented to Her Majesty.

Our homoeopathic cause has the enormous privilege of having The Queen as patron of The Royal London Homoeopathic Hospital. May I, on behalf of all homoeopathic doctors and patients, pay tribute to our Royal Family, who for three generations have given their encouragement and support to homoeopathy.

The Challenge of Homoeopathy

The Patient, Not the Cure

MARGERY G. BLACKIE
Former Physician to Her Majesty, The Queen

London
UNWIN PAPERBACKS
Boston   Sydney

First published in Great Britain by
Macdonald & Jane's as *The Patient, Not the Cure* 1976
Reprinted twice
First published in Unwin Paperbacks 1981

UNWIN® PAPERBACKS
40 Museum Street, London WC1A 1LU

Edited by Felix Brunner

British Library Cataloguing in Publication Data

Blackie, Margery Grace
   The challenge of homoeopathy.
   1. Homoeopathy
   I. Title
   615'.532   RX71   80–41134

   ISBN 0–04–613042–X

Reproduced, printed and bound in Great Britain by
Hazell Watson & Viney Ltd, Aylesbury, Bucks

This book is dedicated to my friend
and partner of over thirty years
the late Dr Helena F. Banks

Contents

Acknowledgements

To Dr Martyn Lloyd-Jones, M.D., M.R.C.P., my grateful thanks for his kindness in sparing the time to read the proofs of this book. Dr Frank Bodman, M.D., F.F.Hom., is due my special thanks for his helpfulness in providing information for one of the chapters and for all his encouragement. My great gratitude goes to Dr Anita Davies, M.B., B.S., M.R.C.P., M.F.Hom., for all the time she gave me and her great help in researching references and articles. I would also like to thank Alan Askew, M.B., Ch.B.Sheff., M.F.Hom., of Sheffield and Dr R. A. F. Jack, M.B., Ch. B. Birm., M.R.C.G.P., M.F.Hom., of Bromsgrove for their advice and encouragement. Also I would like to thank Mr J. B. L. Ainsworth of A. Nelson & Co., Ltd., the homoeopathic pharmacy, for all the trouble he took in looking up tables, and for his generous advice and information. My deep gratitude is due to my friend, Musette Majendie, C.B.E., for her constant helpfulness and advice during the writing of this book. My gratitude also goes to Felix Brenner for his unstinted help and all the time-consuming advice he freely gave.

But of all the people to whom I owe the most gratitude it is those who appear in this book, my patients and those of my colleagues who have given me such a rewarding life.

Introduction

This book is being written at a time when concepts of modern medicine are changing very rapidly. Homoeopathy is a much misunderstood medical art.

The concepts of modern medicine started in the last decade of the eighteenth century. It was a time of great intellectual and scientific investigation. Hahnemann, the founder of the Homoeopathic principle, was among the first to evolve a method of investigation and experimentation into disease and its treatment in the individual. He had been dissatisfied with the results he had obtained as a practising doctor and he wanted to know why. He began to look into the theories and practice of medicine and to find out why theory did not work out in practice. He studied the origins of the theories which had been put forward and felt that they did not at all fit in with the medical practice of his time. As a result of his reading the history of medicine and enquiring into the methods of practice he noticed that throughout its past the concept of 'like curing like' arose and disappeared from time to time. This seemed to confirm some of his own observations that specific diseases occurred under specific conditions such as he had noticed in the marshes of Hungary and in common occupations throughout Europe. In the course of his investigations he found that he disagreed with the application of a certain remedy which was promulgated by the leading therapeutic authority. This started him off on testing drugs on himself, his family, his colleagues and his friends provided they were all in excellent health. More and more Hahnemann, and later his pupils and colleagues, came to recognize over the course of years that no single symptom was sufficient to specify for its cure. This convinced them that it was only by studying the whole man in all his aspects that they could understand the nature and cure of the disease in the individual; that it was indeed the patient and not the cure.

Throughout the history of medicine there is a tendency to treat diseases by methods which were applied to people en masse. Hahnemann's homoeopathic principle is to treat the individual in order to bring the whole man back to his true state of health.

I

Concepts in
Homoeopathy

In his *Principles and Practice of Homoeopathy* Dr Wheeler, one of the finest of English homoeopathic doctors, wrote that very few of those who condemned the practice of homoeopathy had any knowledge of its principles, to say nothing of its practice, and that therefore it is fair to say that in a Court of Science their testimony, however voluble and dogmatic, must be considered invalid.

Hahnemann and his followers made definite statements concerning the use of drugs for the relief of disease, and claimed that their findings were based on clinical experiments which had been repeated many times. These experiments have been continuing for more than 170 years and have been checked and rechecked many times.

Homoeopaths are determined to demonstrate that diseases are made known by their symptoms and signs in the patient. Symptoms here being objective signs, that is physical signs in the patient; and that without the presence of these symptoms or signs an individual cannot be said to be diseased.

Symptom complexes can be produced by administering remedies (drugs) to a healthy person. These symptoms, in most cases, are those which are found to occur in a certain illness. Even in the time of Hippocrates it was noted that if one compared the symptoms of a diseased person with those reactions which were caused by certain drugs in a healthy person that there was a remarkable resemblance between the two. This is the basis of homoeopathy: the most successful drug for administering to the ill is that very drug which produces the same symptoms in someone who is well. Thus the *similimum*, the most resembling drug, should be given: 'Like should be treated by like.' Homoeopathy is therefore a rule of practice for the administration of drugs. It demands a thorough knowledge of the effects of drugs on the healthy and their effectiveness on the diseased.

The successful practice of homoeopathy depends on taking advantage of every opportunity to see it working. There are simple remedies which anyone can use. There are remedies easy to take for all ages, remedies made into powders, tablets or tinctures with no unpleasant taste. There are high potency remedies which can be taken in one dose or three or four doses in one day which are sufficient to start a patient on the road to recovery. Then there are low potency remedies which are prescribed more often on local symptoms, and can be given three or four times a day until improvement sets in. One does not get, nor does one expect, the dramatic effects which one would see after a high potency remedy. Also, low potencies can be taken for three or four weeks if needed. But to do this successfully requires a thorough knowledge of the remedy and the significance of the patient's symptoms. And to do this, one must have been thoroughly trained in medical diagnosis and pathology.

The creed of homoeopathy was so well stated by Hahnemann:

1. The physician's high and *only* mission is to restore the sick to health; to cure, as it is termed.

2. The highest ideal of cure is a rapid, gentle and permanent restoration to health or the removal and total annihilation of the disease in the shortest, most reliable and most harmless way based on easily comprehensible principles. A physician clearly perceives what is to be cured in each individual case because he has learned to identify the symptoms. The doctor clearly perceives what curative medicine is indicated because of his knowledge of the effectiveness of the medicines.

3. According to the well defined principles of diagnosis and pathology, he must know how to adapt the curative treatment for the individual morbid condition of the patient. And to ensure that gentle, rapid and permanent recovery will ensue, he must adapt the preparations, quantity and frequency of the suitable remedy.

4. And finally, if he is aware of the obstacles to recovery and how to remove them, then he understands how to treat judiciously, and is a true practitioner of the healing art. He has become a preserver of health by knowing those things that derange health and cause disease; he knows how to keep a person in health.

To select the right drug is the important thing, and that is done, as we have said, by matching the patient's symptoms and signs with a 'drug picture'—getting the similimum. From Hahnemann's time the search for the similima has been conducted by extensive research and experimentation. And these experiments have been repeated over and over again on groups of volunteers. These volunteers were given drugs whose name and nature were unknown to them. They then noted all the symptoms produced, some of major importance and others trivial, but nevertheless recorded so that from the overall picture thus obtained it was possible to give the range of the drug effects.

Having accumulated all this knowledge of drugs, how have the homoeopaths put them to practical use? Hahnemann had only a very limited *materia medica*, but even so, when he met a sick patient with symptoms which matched those of some drug which he had been testing, he would then prescribe this drug in a small dose. In some patients the symptoms at first increased before there was any response. He then tried giving progressively smaller and smaller doses. He always advocated prescribing the smallest possible dose necessary to help the patient. Being a chemist he knew that the most effective liquid preparations were those in which the mixture was homogeneous. He evolved a method of mixing, diluting and shaking which he called succussion. The result of this was a preparation which, because of its powers, he named a potency. The means of producing this potency were roughly the following: once having created a powder from a mineral source by crushing it between a mortar and pestle, he rendered it liquid by dissolving it in a mixture of alcohol and water; this is called the mother tincture, known as Q from the Greek letter φ. This in turn is further diluted methodically so that one drop of the tincture in nine drops of the diluent is called a 1x, whereas one drop of the tincture in ninety-nine of the diluent is known as a 1c. By a further series of dilution and succussion higher potencies were produced which could go up to any level required. Then it was found that the greater the degree of dilution the more powerful the medicine. And although chemical analysis did not reveal any trace of the original drug in the suspension, the preparation was found to produce a 'symptom picture' corresponding to the proving made on a healthy subject.

Ever since the eighteenth century chemists have been trying to establish the efficacy of medicines by identifying and isolating their chemical components. It has been found, for instance, that the chemical composition of the juices of the leaves of cabbage and Belladonna were identical. And yet the nutritive value of the one is diametrically the opposite of the poisonous effects of the other on humans.

More and more it has become the practice in orthodox medicine to treat the various symptoms in a patient singly; for each complaint a specific medication. And even more frequently various mixtures are assembled in the theory that they will act severally on the patient and that time will be saved. This polypharmacy is far from the Hahnemann principle of the *single* remedy and the similimum which will suit the patient's complaints.

Plants, of course, contain an enormous amount of alkaloids and chemical substances. Today the chemical pharmacist tries to extract what is called 'the active ingredient' which contains the curative principle. But to the homoeopathist this isolated ingredient is of no importance at all since he has 'proved' the entire plant extract and knows the 'symptom picture' it produces, and therefore what illness it cures.

Until now science has been unable to measure what happens when a substance is rendered into a potency. When potentization can be precisely defined perhaps then other methods of preparation may be found which will be as effective as the time proved succussion technique. But until then the time honoured methods of trituration (rendered by crushing in a mortar) and succussion (dilution, mixing and shaking) are the only ones that have been found effective in the nearly two hundred year history of homoeopathic medicine.

The reaction in animals is different from that in humans. And so it is that provings and remedy experimentation is done only on people. This does not prevent us from observing the effects of some of our medicines on animals. Sometimes we have found pathological changes in the tissues of animals where our provings on humans have not extended so far as to reveal them.

The benefit of proving medicines on healthy people is the perfectly obvious one; that they can record all their symptoms, which is something no animal can do. It is from these human records that we learn the reactions in the organism that are both physical and mental. Whereas the testing of active ingredients in animals gives us only a superficial outline of what may be only a relief of a painful symptom with no record of any other distressful side effects.

There is a phrase peculiar to homoeopathy; the Constitutional drug, and for those who are new to homoeopathy I will try to explain it. We sometimes talk of someone having a strong constitution, but what does that mean? According to *Chambers' Encyclopaedia* the original definition is 'fundamental system of laws governing the body'. This is in terms of our medical, physiological body, but beyond that we are individual: each of us has our own personality and our own characteristic ways of acting. The constitutional drug is that which is most effective in treating the individual in the sum total of his strengths and weaknesses; mentally, emotionally and physically.

A man pre-eminent in the field of orthodox medicine, Lord Cohen of Birkenhead, has often repeated, 'We must return to the study of the whole man. Increasing specialization in practice has led to increased compartmentalism, departmentalism and fragmentation in teaching, with all the evils that follow. The doctor must never forget that man is more than the sum of his parts. Basic medical teaching must aim at presenting a "synoptic" view of man, in health and in disease. Unless this be achieved, then the training will be misdirected in aim, in structure and in balance. The student will lack the necessary guiding principles when confronted with the novel situations which rear daily in front of him in typical practice.'

This point of view is further expanded in *Symptoms and Their Interpretations* by Sir James McKenzie:

> ... the general practitioners are the people who are brought into contact with the illnesses which impair the health of the community. An analysis of the complaints which the general practitioner sees reveals the present state of medical knowledge. If we put aside the trivial ailments, and consider the illnesses which lower the health of the great majority of people, it is found that only a small percentage (5–10%) are capable of being diagnosed with any degree of accuracy. Most of this small percentage are cases of disease so advanced that the organs are damaged beyond repair ... the end result of a long period of bad health, but the origin of the ill health was not detectable.

He goes on to say 'many valuable signs are only perceptible to the trained eye, or the trained ear, or the trained finger. Still more valuable signs are only revealed by the sensations experienced by the patient'. He also wrote that, 'Few attempts are made to train men for the detection of ... disease when there is a hope of cure.' and that 'The early stages are, as a rule, insidious, and are indicated mainly by subjective sensation.' All of this might have been written by a homoeopath, for it is these early signs and symptoms that direct us to the constitutional remedy. Trousseau put it another way: 'There are no diseases; there are only ill people.'

And so it is in the early, undiagnosable stages of illness that we must find the constitutional drug. You must study the patients; how do they look?; how do they behave?; what are they saying? It is much easier to assess the child who isn't quite ill, but just feels not himself than it is with an adult. Time, circumstance, education, opinions, self-control all enter into the picture and so it needs extra effort until you can discern the real person. And until a bit of information is revealed that had been even innocently withheld, we can be thwarted in our attempt to find the constitutional drug.

One of my colleagues had a patient who suffered acutely from arthritis and for whom everything, including cortisone, had been prescribed, all without success. He was still running a high temperature, and was very ill and so exhausted that he had no reaction to anything. Fortunately for the doctor—and for him—soon after he was admitted to hospital the weather changed and we were having a heat wave. Not long later one of his nurses complained angrily that the patient was quite impossible in demanding attention all day and all night. She hadn't the staff to cope with his whims. When the physician went to visit him he found a changed man. 'This heat,' he said, 'I can't bear it.' The doctor reminded him that he had lived for years in Ceylon and thought he rather liked warm weather. But the patient replied that this was all different 'no air stirring at all'. He was irritable under the stress of the heat, and wanted help, sympathy and attention; and it was this reaction that revealed his true constitution. He was given a high potency of *Pulsatilla* which lowered his temperature the next day and he was well on the way to recovery. Had it not been for the stress aggravation the doctor would never have known the real man.

Hippocrates, called the Father of Medicine, is credited with saying that Nature is the curer of diseases. This was the base on which Hahnemann and homoeopathic doctors have established their creed in their determination to help nature and not to fight it.

2

Hahnemann the Man

In order to understand homoeopathy one has to look back to its history. It was first fully recognized by Dr Samuel Hahnemann although he realized that it had been mentioned by Hippocrates and again by Paracelsus. But it was Hahnemann who investigated it in a very long series of experiments. The veracity and intelligence of the man who did this work is beyond dispute and I have tried to show in this brief account of Hahnemann the man something of his great character and training.

It has often been said that homoeopathy existed before Hahnemann. So it did; in the same way as gravity existed before Newton.

The phrase *similia similibus curentur* (like will be cured by like) occurs repeatedly in medical treatises from the most ancient of times. And in the sixteenth and seventeenth centuries the question of whether diseases are best cured by similars or by contraries arises with increasing frequency. In his endeavour to perfect the art of medicine Hahnemann had delved so deeply in the literature of chemistry and medicine that it is difficult to tell whether he had borrowed the idea of the *similia* from the ancients or had worked it out himself. However, Dr Compton-Burnett, the famous lecturer on homoeopathy, having himself investigated the matter thoroughly (so thoroughly in fact that he nearly doubted the originality of Hahnemann's theory) finally came to the conclusion that the German doctor had evolved his own system.

Until Hahnemann came to his conclusions and put his concepts of homoeopathy into a system there had been, since the time of Paracelsus, several other 'methods' of homoeopathic treatments. One of these was entitled the Doctrine of Signature. This theory was reasoned on the lines of similarity: Thus the juice of *Chelidonium* (celandine) which is yellow must be the cure for bad bile since the bile is yellow. In a like manner since the meat of the walnut resembles the brain it must be good for the brain. Another was based on the universe, known as the macrocosm, and the body of man, known as the microcosm. Every part of the universe had its component part in man. So the sun, the heart of the universe and glowing with the colour of gold, gives the name sol to the metal as part of the macrocosm. In the microcosm man, the heart is sol and so gold is the remedy for cardiac conditions. Then there was the obvious likeness of the parts of animals to the parts of man. So pulmonary diseases and even asthma should be treated by the lungs of foxes. (This, incidentally, was a very popular and long-lived theory.) A fourth idea held that certain types of disease prevail in certain regions of the world and that in these regions, or those similar to them, there are specific remedies to be found. Since *Solanum dulcamara* (bittersweet) is found in a cold damp place it must be the cure for chills, just as aches and pains are helped by *Salix* (willow) which grows in the damp and soggy areas which are the breeding grounds of rheumatic conditions.

Unquestionably Hahnemann had read these and other theories. With all their divergencies they were still a source of inspiration in allowing him to analyse, investigate, experiment and reject until he began to find the means to formulate his law of healing. And as these experiments progressed it became apparent to him that this law was going to be based on *similia similibus curentur*. It was experiments on himself in investigating the properties of *Cinchona* (quinine) that convinced him.

Christian Friedrich Samuel Hahnemann was born in Meissen in 1755. His parents were people of education and taste, but extremely poor. While still a young boy his mind was shaped by his father who would set the child a problem and then put him in a room on his own and give him time to think it out. He thus developed a faculty for concentration which, despite many vicissitudes later enabled him to take up the study of medicine. His father's profession was that of a painter on porcelain. The political conditions of the mid 1760s severely cut short the demand for fine china and the boy had to be apprenticed to a grocer, cutting short his school career. Fortunately the rector of the school recognized the waste and persuaded the elder Hahnemann to let the boy return to his studies without having to pay school fees. Samuel was the pet of the rector who devoted some of his spare time to further his education. By the time he was thirteen Hahnemann was sufficiently skilful to give his fellow pupils lessons in Hebrew. When he went to Leipzig, to study medicine, at the age of twenty, he was already an accomplished linguist. He had no money to speak of, but his ability to translate scientific works enabled him to make a living whilst he was training. Since he was proficient in eight languages his work was much in demand, but he confined his money making time to working on his translations every third night. This habit of devoting his energies to his studies and life work, interrupted by writing at specific times, endured for forty years. And it is this habit which explains his prolific literary output. He managed to save enough money to leave Leipzig for Vienna to study at the most advanced school of medicine in Europe. He was an exceptional young man whose diligence and willingness endeared him to his teachers, and especially to his Professor. He took the young man under his own care and treated him like a son.

While still a student Hahnemann became family physician and librarian to the Governor of Transylvania. In his course of duty with the governor he spent two years in the all but impenetrable marshy lands of lower Hungary. The area was notorious for the number of people suffering from ague with all the concomitant ailments of that condition. By the time he qualified, when he was just over twenty-four, he acquired a thorough knowledge of the illness and the treatments for it. He did not cease to translate for scientific publishers so that during the whole of his medical curriculum he was able to pay his own way and earn a living. He was, we know, a prodigious worker who found time to make the most use of what he had learned in Leipzig and Vienna.

In 1782, while serving as medical officer of health in Gommern, a small town near Magdeburg, he married the daughter of an apothecary. Their life together was a happy one despite the many changes of home and the controversies he caused in the medical profession. They had been married but two years when they moved on to Dresden. With his friendly ways and thoroughness he soon established himself in his profession and translation work. Then in 1786, when Hahnemann was but 31, his great admirer, the chief surgeon of the city, fell ill and the young man from Meissen was asked to take his place. By that time he had an exceptional reputation throughout Germany not only as a doctor but as an author and a chemist. Among the many articles he published, one was a study on Arsenical Poisoning which was dedicated to 'The Majesty of the Good Kaiser Joseph'.

During the next few years his reputation was further enhanced by his co-operation with other members of the medical profession and his work side by side with chemists experimenting in their laboratories, so that he had made a name for himself in the worlds of medicine and of science. His literary labours had carried his fame far beyond the confines of his country and had already captured the attention of his colleagues. The more he investigated contemporary theories and practices the more his doubts increased as to the benefit of medical treatments. By the end of the century he was not alone in believing that current medicine was not only not good, but positively harmful. The most unscientific and complicated prescriptions were applied indiscriminately; patients were bled by venesection and cupping, and leeches by the dozen were applied to those suffering from any complaint from tuberculosis to colic. His discontent was mirrored in the writings of Sir John Forbes: 'In a considerable proportion of diseases, it would fare well, or better, for the patients if all remedies were abandoned. . . . Things have arrived at such a pitch that they cannot be worse. They must mend or end.' With all his doubts Hahnemann continued in his practice and in his research. To Sir John he was one of the few lights in a dismal prospect when he wrote of him, '. . . no candid observer of his actions or writings would hesitate for a moment to admit that he was a very extraordinary man, a man of genius and a scholar; a man of indefatigable industry and of dauntless energy.' Hufeland, who was a leading German physician, and publisher of the most scientific medical journal of the time, speaks of him as one of the most distinguished physicians in Germany, and published Hahnemann's articles in his paper. Despite his fame, by 1796 Hahnemann was in despair. With all his knowledge of orthodox methods, and with all his experimentation along those lines his results were very disappointing. He all but gave up his practice and devoted more and more of his time earning a living by translating foreign medical books into German. And then, suddenly, while working on a translation of Cullen's *Materia Medica*, he had an experience which was to change his thinking and, as a result, his life.

William Cullen, who had died only six years earlier, at the age of eighty, had been a most distinguished Scottish physician. He was Professor of Medicine at Glasgow for five years until 1755 and from then until the end of his days he was at Edinburgh. His fame was extensive and he was considered the leading authority on the therapeutics practised and recommended during the last part of the eighteenth century. But, while working on the translation of Cullen's *Materia Medica*, Hahnemann found himself disagreeing utterly with the famous Scotsman's explanation of the action of quinine in the treatment of malaria. He then decided to test the drug on himself, and here he had a stroke of good fortune such as blesses the Isaac Newtons and the Howard Floreys in the world of science.

Hahnemann found that he was sensitive to quinine; not that he was allergic to it, but that he had a definite idiosyncracy or reaction, to it. He found that after taking a dose of quinine he was soon suffering from the symptoms of an illness similar to those he had frequently seen as a medical student in the marshlands of lower Hungary. In short, except for the fever, he was experiencing the symptoms of malaria. It then occurred to him that if this drug could produce symptoms similar to those of malaria, it then, might be the cure for malaria. It is then that he first applied the words to his theory, *similia similibus curentur*: Like will be cured by like, which is the slogan of the homoeopath.

His experience of twenty years told him that he had to test his theory. Like every true scientist he decided to concentrate on producing evidence to prove or disprove his new-found conclusion. He set out to experiment with other substances; and for twenty years he continued to investigate the action of substances on healthy people. He recruited himself, his family, his friends and volunteers from among medical students. The drugs were always given singly, never in combination, so that whatever the effect of the drug taken, it could be only from that one particular drug. Each volunteer had to be healthy. They were not allowed to smoke, to drink brandy, wine, tea or coffee and they were prohibited from taking pepper, ginger or strongly salted foods. To ensure that the volunteers were accurately recording any and all symptoms or sensations, they were denied the distractions of billiards, cards or chess. Above all, the volunteers were never told what substance it was that they were proving. Hahnemann was rigorous in examining the reports of his volunteers, or 'provers' as they were called, and each had to carry a notebook and pencil to record any reactions which occurred as they happened and when they happened. He examined and cross-examined his helpers to make sure that they had put down their sensations without any exaggeration.

By the time he published his *Materia Medica* in 1810 he had collected information on sixty-seven remedies some known to medicine and some unknown. Each substance was investigated and for each one every symptom, major or minor was recorded. This series of reactions gave him a total picture of the effects of each drug. At the same time he expounded his theories on his findings in the *Organon der Rationellen Heilkunde* (*The Classification of Practical*

Medicines) in which for the first time he defined the creed, method and role of homoeopathic medicine.

With the publication of his two books Hahnemann didn't stop his tireless search for verification or rejection of his theories. Doubtless he was having successes with isolated cases, but these were not really enough to test his findings to the full. Once again the time was ripe. Three years later the terrible winter of 1812 took its toll of Napoleon's army in Russia. The bedraggled remnants of the Grande Armée were staggering, starving, bleeding and riddled with disease while drifting across Europe on their way home. Despite their desperate condition the French fought valiantly, but lost the three-day battle at Leipzig in August 1813. The aftermath was not only death but a fearful epidemic of typhoid. At once Hahnemann put his hypothesis to the test. He treated 180 cases and his success bordered on the miraculous: only one patient died. Now his fame spread throughout Europe.

Two years later he became unpaid lecturer in medicine at the University of Leipzig, a post which he held for six years. Toward the end of his tenure he ran into serious trouble with the apothecaries of the city. For some time he had been having difficulty in acquiring the necessary medicines for the treatment of his patients. Desperate to improve matters he not only prescribed his tinctures, powders and tablets, but made and dispensed them himself. The wrath of the pharmaceutical chemists was too much and they had their revenge. Hahnemann could no longer withstand their prejudices and retired to the town of Cöthen (now Köthen) quietly working for several years.

Hahnemann published his *Materia Medica* because it was obvious to him that a lexicon or dictionary of symptoms was needed. All the original experiments were repeated in healthy people who were called provers. The expected reaction of the drug on the majority of the provers was recognized as a symptom characteristic. Now, when an unhealthy person exhibited these same symptom characteristics and was treated with the drug these symptoms disappeared. Gradually Hahnemann accumulated data which he assembled in such an order that the 'keynotes' of the particular characteristic symptoms of each remedy were separated from the hundreds of recorded symptoms. Further classification became possible and Hahnemann himself noticed that certain physical and mental constitutions reacted in almost predictable ways when prescribed a particular medicine; whereas with similar symptoms, but with a different physical and mental makeup, the response to the medicine was different. Hahnemann also held that in the body there was a self-preserving, self-balancing mechanism that kept it in health in spite of the stress and strain to which man is subject. The body's nervous system and its ductless glands, such as the suprarenals, automatically prepare it for any undue stress, and with very little assistance from a doctor. For instance, a normal body temperature is maintained despite the extremities of weather; and a stable chemical balance is maintained despite our food and fluid consumption. But when too much stress is put upon it, whether it be physical, mental or bacterial, or should the balance normally maintained become impaired, then abnormal signs and symptoms occur and the health becomes upset.

Until the homoeopathic doctors conducted experiments on the effects of medicine the only comparable study was one that was made on the prevention of scurvy. Captain James Cook proved during the three year voyage to Australia (1772–1775) that he could prevent the outbreak of the fatal disease with a diet which included fresh fruit and vegetables. This was a controlled experiment: those who kept to the diet did not succumb and those without the fresh vegetables developed bleeding gums and all the other symptoms of the malady. Despite the obvious benefits the experiment made patent to all who could see, the sailors were all but mutinous in their reluctance to change their diet. Not until the officers were observed to be eating fresh cabbage and chewing on lemons would the lower deck change their ways.

In building up his *Materia Medica* Hahnemann came across another discovery. He found that the provings of *Belladonna* presented all the signs and symptoms of scarlet-fever. In a time of an epidemic of the fever he prescribed the drug with spectacular results which revealed an interesting side-effect. There was a family, every member of which succumbed to scarlet-fever except one child who had been given *Belladonna* previously. *Belladonna* clearly not only cures scarlet-fever but can act as a prophylactic against it when the infection is around.

The general therapeutic medicines of his day were put to the same experimentations by Hahnemann and his colleagues. But at the same time he looked around in the industrial workshops and noted the toxic effects upon the workers when in constant contact with mercury, arsenic and sulphur, among others. He tested all these substances on his healthy volunteers and discovered much about their action which was of value in the treatment of sick people. Experiments were also conducted using inert substances such as gold, copper and silica which were insoluble. Hahnemann was the first to render these soluble by trituration; that is by pounding and pulverising the inert substance and mixing it in a combination of alcohol and water. Thus he produced what came to be known as colloidal solutions.

In 1831 Hahnemann was able once again to test and prove his theories in a massive way. This time all of Europe came down with an epidemic of cholera. Between

June and October of that year Hahnemann published at no fee for himself four pamphlets on the treatment of the infection. These were widely circulated in Leipzig and Berlin. One of his pupils put the hypothesis to practical application in Leipzig and treated 154 victims homoeopathically. He lost six, whereas the orthodox doctors, treating some 1500 patients, lost 821. In other towns doctors acting on Hahnemann's principles had equal success.

The *Organon der Rationellen Heilkunde*, first published in 1810 went through five editions before Hahnemann died in 1843. And as each edition succeeded the other his ideas were developed. His three requirements of a good physician were that he find out: What it is in the patient that requires help; What are the means by which he can help his patient; That he apply his knowledge in restoring the patient to full health and enable him to enjoy a full life.

As the work progressed from edition to edition some of his concepts changed. At first he considered the symptoms occurring in the patient as signs that the body was attempting to heal itself, and so true therapy should encourage this. However he later learned how very inept nature can be in trying to cure itself and so he further expanded his views on the function of therapy in disease. He used the term 'vital force' to describe the balancing mechanism in every living body which promotes, or at least protects, health. He wrote that this 'vital force' was stimulated by internal and external disorders to build up a reaction to counteract the disorders. The result of the interaction between the 'vital force' and the conditions which set it in motion produces various symptoms in the body revealing that an imbalance has occurred. And it is these symptoms which the physician notices and which should tell him which medicine is most likely to cure the patient. Thus a disease can be considered a product of stress and the failure of the body's own attempts to overcome it. The advances in techniques of investigation and analysis since Hahnemann's day have confirmed the picture he had drawn so vividly. To-day it is widely recognized that a rheumatic disorder may result from an over-responsive immunizing reaction within the body. A build up of the counteracting agent, known today as an antibody, will then follow. This causes damage to other cells and proteins and creates even more tissue damage. This illustrates Hahnemann's concept of 'inept Nature'. For example it is not unusual for someone to have been inoculated against whooping cough and to succumb to the infection if he comes in contact with the organism when it is virulent enough.

In time Hahnemann found that living in Cöthen kept him too inaccessible to those living outside Germany who wished to consult with him. His fame had spread across the Channel and his British colleagues and admirers had their work made more difficult because of the time it took for letters to go and come. In any event he felt that the more congenial intellects of the French would help in the dissemination of his work and theories. Accordingly he moved to Paris in 1835. Once installed he was consulted by doctors, chemists and scientists from all over Europe until he died eight years later.

The first homoeopathic physicians had to rely solely on the patient's symptoms when trying to prescribe a remedy. They had no aids to diagnosis such as bacteriological analyses, blood chemistry, urine analysis or other means of detection. What they relied on then, and still do, is the totality of symptoms. For them it is essential that they do not select one sympton which a patient may display and match that with one similar symptom in the effect of the drug. The whole history of the patient's symptoms must be matched against the whole picture of the *similimum*, the nearest drug picture.

The business of successfully prescribing homoeopathically is very exciting and very rewarding. Because, once the one and only *similimum* is identified, and once it has been prescribed there is no doubt in the mind of the patient or of the doctor. What greater reward is there than the enormous satisfaction of making someone really better and happier and able to carry on his work?

Hahnemann's work and writings were not only concerned with the medical and pharmaceutical practices of his contemporaries. He was adamantly against the appalling treatment given the insane. He was appalled at the chastisements, the blows and beatings these unfortunates suffered; he was horrified at the overcrowded conditions in the institutions with their concomitant dirt, lack of fresh air, and unsanitariness. 'The physician in charge of such unhappy people,' he said, 'must have at his command an attitude which inspires respect and creates confidence.' In line with this thinking he advocated the building of isolation hospitals against the time of epidemics and a spacious town planning with houses in gardens set in wide streets to afford air and proper sanitation for all.

Hahnemann was not alone in recognizing the shortcomings of medical practice and theory in his time; but he was in the forefront of those who, in a society plagued with epidemic, sought the swiftest, gentlest and most permanent means for the restoration and preservation of health.

3

Contemporaries of Hahnemann

England's first practising homoeopathic doctor was Frederick Foster Hervey Quin. His early history is extremely obscure, all that we do know is that he was born in 1799. His name suggests that he was a grandson of the famous Earl-Bishop of Bristol, Frederick Augustus Hervey. He went to Mr Trimmer's school in Putney and as soon as the Battle of Waterloo was won in 1815 he was sent to Paris to learn French. By the end of fifteen months he was reputed to speak the language better than he did English. In 1817 he was studying medicine at the University of Edinburgh and in three years he qualified as a doctor. His graduation thesis was on Arsenic, a very topical subject, as the new science of chemistry was the current fashion.

At that time a young doctor embarking on a professional career needed a patron. Sir Hudson Lowe, governor of St Helena was attacked for his rigorous surveillance of Napoleon by the ex-Emperor's British doctor, Barry Edward O'Meara. There were charges and counter-charges on both sides, each blaming the other for the prisoner's ill health. Questions were raised in Parliament, and the Prime Minister, Lord Liverpool, appointed the newly qualified Dr Quin to be physician in attendance on the exiled Emperor. However before he embarked for St Helena in the summer of 1821 news arrived of the Emperor's death.

Quin's health, even at this early stage, was very poor and friends urged foreign travel as a possible remedy. He had only to wait six months when he was invited to visit Italy with the Duchess of Devonshire as her medical attendant. The position had the marked advantage that in her company he had ample opportunity to see the great world of places and persons. As in Hahnemann's case when appointed to the Governor of Transylvania, Quin's duties were not only medical. By the summer the Duchess no longer required his constant attendance and Quin removed to Naples determined to set up in practice there. He had an agreement with his patroness that should she need him he would go to her whenever required. Despite being plagued with headaches and ill health, his medical practice became extensive and he soon numbered Sir William Hamilton, Sir William Gell and Sir Henry Drummond among his close friends.

The next year was spent largely between attending to the Duchess, who by then was living 16 miles to the south-east of Naples, and establishing his practice and friendships in Naples. In July 1823 he received an invitation to join Byron as his physician in the forthcoming expedition to help the Greek rebels. He was sorely tempted, and was urged to go by his protector. But he was having too much trouble with his lung condition and in the end he decided that the journey would be too hazardous. He wrote to the Duchess of his determination to stay in Naples and she replied 'God bless you, my dear sir; may your success be equal to my good wishes, and I have no doubt of it. There are always some difficulties to beginners but you will soon get over all these.' Quin unquestionably combined great charm and close aristocratic connections with ability and as his popularity increased so did his practice.

In the spring of 1824 Quin had his first contact with homoeopathy when his friend William Gell wrote him from Rome. Sir William suffered from gout and wrote to his friend that he was being treated by a Dr George Necker who was a disciple of Hahnemann's. Later that year Quin made a hurried visit to England and Scotland. Upon his return to Italy in December he met Thomas Uwins, an encounter which became the foundation of a lifelong friendship.

In the following year he met Dr Necker. It came about just as he was becoming interested in works on homoeopathy. Necker was invaluable in putting him in touch with much of the literature on the subject. Quin decided to investigate this new system only after most careful consideration of its theories. He then determined to give up his practice for a while and seek information at headquarters. And so it was that he found himself in Leipzig in July 1826, having travelled there by way of Venice, Trieste and Vienna.

He wrote to Thomas Uwins, who had been living in his house in Naples for some months: '. . . I do not wish to appear before the world either as a disciple of, or opponent to, Hahnemann until I feel myself fully competent to do justice to the side which I may ultimately be conscientiously induced to take. Although my principal object has been to get acquainted with Hahnemann's opinions and practice I have not neglected to get all the information I possibly could of the state of medicine and the hospitals in Germany. I have worked most laboriously, and can really say that I have picked up a great deal of valuable information in my profession, laying aside altogether the new system, so that whatever it may turn out to be, I have managed so as never to allow myself to regret having come to Germany. I have several times been very much disheartened, and very doubtful of the propriety of my undertaking owing to conversation with the different professors, who laughed at the very idea of an English physician thinking of studying such a system . . . as they are all men of talent, information and reputation in their profession . . . but on pushing my questions further I found that some had never read the books of Hahnemann, and that not one had put the system to the test, not one had tried the effect of the medicines . . . not one had proved the truth or fallacy of the system by experiment. Very little reflection convinced me that no weight was to be given to opinions which rested upon prejudices arising from their previous education.'

On the day he wrote this letter he succumbed to another inflammation of his lungs which nearly proved fatal. Yet three weeks later he was able to write to his friend:

'. . . I was seized with most violent pains in the chest, great oppression of breath, violent cough, expectoration of bloody mucus and blood, great anxiety, and fear of suffocation, so much so as to make me and my physician think that I would not recover. . . . I myself, however am a living proof of the efficacy of the new system. I have had in my life three inflammatory attacks on the lungs, all of them sufficiently violent, but none more dangerous nor equal to this; indeed I never saw one with more dangerous symptoms. I used to be purged, sweated, blistered and bled, the latter enormously; in my last illness . . . it was thought necessary to take as much as one hundred and twenty five ounces of blood. In this illness I have not taken a single purge, no soporifics, no blisters and have not lost one drop of blood . . . and everything that my physician told me as to the probable effect of the different medicines they gave me came to pass. I only took five small powders, which had no other taste but that of sugar. . . . What annoys me most is my not being allowed to pursue my studies. . . .'

His recuperation took six weeks, but by mid-November he went to Naumberg to visit Dr Stapf, the editor of the *Homoeopathic Journal* and from there went to study a week or ten days with Hahnemann in Cöthen. It is a measure of Quin's adaptability that although he had been associated with the dandies of his time he could accommodate himself to Hahnemann's rigid routine. Quin, as usual, endeared himself to the household and kept up a friendship with the founder of homoeopathy until his death. Quin claimed that he was the oldest and favourite English pupil of the Master.

But before he made his calls he fagged away at a most prodigious rate, nine hours of hard reading a day in the hopes of mastering the theory of homoeopathy and learning all he could from others. Other than that he was determined to learn for himself by putting to the test of experiment all the knowledge he had acquired. It was his bad health that he found the greatest drawback; for it prevented him from trying some of the medicines on himself.

Quin was much impressed with what he called the new system, but he had to weigh carefully his decision to practise it when he returned to Naples. He broke his journey homeward from Leipzig in Rome where he met and impressed Prince Leopold of Saxe-Coburg (later to be famous as the first king of the Belgians and Queen Victoria's 'Uncle Leopold'). If, once in Naples, he did not abandon his orthodox medical treatments, he was a staunch defender of Hahnemann's theories as practised by Dr Necker. Far from having his reputation diminished it was increased. Then in the spring of 1827 he was invited by Leopold of Saxe-Coburg to become his physician. He was attached to the royal household with a handsome salary with no restrictive conditions on his practice except that of living at Marlborough House, dining at the Prince's table and travelling with his suite. It was with sadness that he relinquished his practice in Naples and in June he returned to England in the company of his new employer.

The Prince was very low in mental and bodily vigour when they arrived and Quin advised a course of treatment which was opposed by the Prince's other doctor, Baron Stockmar. Quin, a young man of only 26, held his ground, convinced his royal patron and won the day. Stockmar was most kind in writing to the young man telling him how right he had been to urge the Prince to go bathing in the sea. 'His Royal Highness never was so well nor looked better than he did.'

Not long after they returned to London one of the members of the Royal staff was stricken with a disease that all, including Quin, thought fatal. The dying man was treated by a homoeopathic doctor and recovered. This determined Quin in his acceptance of homoeopathy and it is said that from this time he became the first practitioner in Britain. Quin remained a member of the Prince's household for the years 1827 to 1829. When in May 1829 he left his employ he received a letter from Stockmar: 'In acquainting you by command of HRH the Prince Leopold that he is pleased to relieve you from your present duties, I have to add that it is only from the motive of having no longer occasion for a resident medical man in his family. As HRH thinks it might be agreeable to you, your name will be continued amongst the Physicians in Ordinary of the Prince and you are at liberty to wear the uniform of his household.'

But the British climate did not suit him at all physically nor in his practice. He found all opinion against him in his espousal of the Hahnemannian system and upon the advice of friends betook himself to Paris in 1830. His reputation and connections stood him in good stead and soon he was one of the most popular of the English residents in that city. His friendly accord there was tempered with the urge to return to London and fight the bigots ranged against homoeopathy. Again his circle of friends and admirers helped him, and he thus avoided a certain clash not only amongst those of his colleagues in medicine, but a headlong struggle with the Society of Apothecaries. He continued in Paris maintaining a steady correspondence with England. By mid-summer in the following year Europe and England were swept by a new epidemic of cholera. In every country methods were being sought to stem the disease which some thought to be Indian, and not European, in origin. So it was that in September Quin gave up his Parisian practice to consult with Hahnemann and to learn from him what methods he was using in his fight against the epidemic then raging in Germany. He volunteered at once to go to Tischnowitz in Moravia where the disease was endemic. He was barely on the scene when he himself succumbed to an attack. As soon as he was able to crawl he set to work with indomitable energy. The situation was graphically recalled by the mayor of Tischnowitz in his letter of gratitude:

'When the doctor arrived at this place to investigate the cholera epidemic it had reached it highest pitch in the town and the surrounding village of Varkcloster, both as regards the number of victims and the violence of the symptoms, so that often death ensued in a few hours. It happened just at this time the three medical men, Dr Gerstel, Hanesh and Linhart were all ill; although you yourself were struck down immediately upon your arrival, you undertook as soon as convalescent the treatment of the sick, with the greatest readiness and benevolence during the days when Dr Gerstel was obliged to keep to his bed, and with such great success that from that time no patient died. The local authorities consider it their duty to tender their warmest thanks for your generosity accompanied with so much help.'

Quin published his results in French and dedicated the pamphlet to the French King, Louis Philippe:

'I owe my life,' he wrote, 'to the Spirit of Camphor. I was suddenly attacked by cholera when at dinner; without any warning. I lost consciousness. I was immediately carried to bed and as soon as I regained my senses I had recourse to this medicine, and after the sixth dose the cramps, the efforts to vomit, the burning in the stomach, the sinking sensations, the vertigo, the slow heart beats were much diminished. The borborygmi (abdominal rumblings), the colour of face and extremities, this marble colour, yielded with less promptitude, yet disappeared by degrees. Although my sufferings were less violent, in comparison to those one sees in cholera, yet the attack was so sudden that I am convinced that had I not had recourse at once to the spirit of camphor I should have succumbed in a very few hours. For several days following I still had a livid circle around the eyes, a great state of weakness, slight nausea with vertigo, headache, constriction of the chest which compelled me to seek the open air, or to lie down. But I must state that at the time I was overworking from morning to night treating cases of cholera, all the other doctors being bedridden.'

In two months after publishing the pamphlet, July 1832, Quin was installed in London at 19 King Street, and as he had so rightly foretold, his practice soon became extensive. One historian has written of this time in Quin's life: 'Well it was for homoeopathy that it had such an one to be its sponsor. Had a man of no note or position adopted it, it would have won its way by degrees, and slowly perhaps. But with Quin to introduce it to England, it got a firm hold of the highest grades of society first of all . . . Quin's character and prospects were sufficient to dispel from the mind of every one who knew him the idea that he adopted homoeopathy from any other motive than that which was inspired by a conviction of its truth. From the first he resolved to maintain the highest professional tone towards his opponents. . . .'

His popularity and success were such that he was soon under attack in some medical journals which denounced him as a quack, an imposter or a charlatan. The outcry of his enemies was so severe that at one point he was challenged by the Censors of the Royal College of Physicians as to the legality of his practising in London, or within seven miles of the city. He ignored this and answered a following note to the effect that he hadn't replied to the first one since he didn't think the situation applied to him. The matter was dropped. However, because of the man's sense of humour, evident conviction and reputation for integrity, Quin was generally on the best of terms with the more advanced thinking of his colleagues in medicine. There were, of course, many who would oppose him no matter how blindly. When in 1838 Quin was put up for membership at the Athenaeum Club his nomination was bitterly opposed by Dr Paris, the president of the Royal College of Physicians. Upon noting Quin's name in the application book he abused Quin to his friends, calling him a quack and imposter and stated that he intended to blackball him. The next day Quin put his situation to Lord Clarence Paget, a son of his friend the Marquis of Anglesey, who immediately took the matter into his own hands. Quin's friend surprised the offensive Dr Paris and demanded a written apology or to justify his language with pistols at twelve paces. The note Paris duly gave was deemed not sufficient and Lord Clarence Paget insisted on a fuller apology, which he in due course received. Notwithstanding, Paris won the day, for Quin received forty-four blackballs, an unheard of number. But Quin and his friends treated the result in a light hearted manner returning vindictive scorn with good humour.

But it was the only time in his long career that he took any notice of the personal attacks. He was scrupulous in giving no grounds for complaint in medical etiquette. He never attempted to answer any attack on himself in the papers or medical journals. For several years he refused fees for medical advice, and to avoid the accusation of writing popular books he had his scientific writings published in French or Latin.

In 1843 Hahnemann died in Paris. It had been the practice of homoeopathic doctors in Germany and France to celebrate his birthday. In the following year Quin invited ten of his colleagues to a dinner at his home to commemorate the founder. And it was at this dinner that he finally, after pondering the idea for seven years, put forth the notion of founding the British Homoeopathic Society.

Dr Quin and many of his colleagues then had to face not only opposition from allopathic doctors but also from some members of the Society. For a time the members were distracted by the differing opinions on forming the laws which were to regulate admission to the Society. Quin had been elected president, and through a voluminous correspondence he never diverged from the duties and course of conduct he thought necessary for the Society. He was determined to uphold its honour and integrity, and in the end, with those fellows and members who agreed with him, he brought the Society triumphantly out of its difficulties.

During the next two years the College of Physicians and Surgeons was urged by many of its members to take action against the homoeopathic doctors, but this they wisely and resolutely refused to do. However, a report on irregular practices was published as a Resolution by the Provincial Medical and Surgical Association in 1846. This 'blast' received a 'counterblast' by Dr Quin in the name of the British Homoeopathic Society. The rebuttal mentioned the widespread legal acceptance of the practice in the United States of America, Bavaria, Baden, other German states, France, Russia and Austria. It further stated that the British Homoeopathic Society either 'through the Press, the Pulpit or the Platform' had never tried in any way to heap contempt upon their allopathic brethren; their conviction being that nothing could tend more to retard their cause than the use of taunts and imputations, in lieu of the calm statement of such evidence as from time to time it was in their power to furnish.

In 1854 there was a severe outbreak of cholera in London. The London Homoeopathic Hospital, then in Golden Square, was converted to the sole treatment of the victims with astonishing results. Nevertheless the Medical Council would not credit the accomplishments and did not report on it in their Blue book, despite the declaration of Dr Maclouchlin, the medical inspector. Quin saw to it that questions were raised in Parliament which resulted in a separate Blue book reporting the London Homoeopathic Hospital's figures. These revealed that where the death rate in other hospitals was 51·8%, in the London Homoeopathic Hospital the rate was only 16·4% in all true cholera cases. The report also read in fact that the medical inspector had seen cases in the Homoeopathic Hospital recover which would have died in other institutions.

After the Crimean War, a new Medical Bill was drafted and again, as ten years earlier, there was a risk that homoeopathic physicians would be disqualified from practice. But Lord Ebury, who as Lord Russell Grosvenor had been Quin's travelling companion twenty years earlier, came to the rescue. At the very last moment as the Bill was being read for the third time in the House of Lords he secured a saving amendment.

It is hard to bear in mind that Dr Quin's immense devotion and energy were constantly besieged by bouts of illness that often rendered him immobile. His health had never been strong but he devoted what remained of his powers to the Homoeopathic Society and the London Homoeopathic Hospital. This dedicated man was also the perfect host and guest, and no dinner party from that of the Prince of Wales down was considered complete without his presence. His perfect manners and his thorough knowledge of human nature made him the pet of society. His tact, sagacity and truthfulness also made him the best of friends. The last eighteen years of his life were wasted away by increasingly severe attacks of asthma, yet he could proudly, and with modesty, say 'I have had my day, I have done my duty, I have realized my ideals . . .'.

Quin's contemporary across the Atlantic was Constantine Hering, who was born 1st January, 1800 at Oschatz in Saxony. He was another who contributed largely to the spread and success of homoeopathy. Even in early childhood he showed a great desire to investigate everything. Being an apt scholar he soon mastered the preliminary studies which enabled him to enter the Classical School at Zittan when he was only eleven. Here he displayed an aptitude for study and gained an accumulation of knowledge far beyond his years by the time he was seventeen. He knew the classics well and had a truly surprising proficiency in mathematics. Then his mind turned to medicine and he took the first opportunity that presented itself to study at the Surgical Academy in Dresden and then later at the University of Leipzig. It was here that he became a pupil of the eminent surgeon, Robbi.

At about this time Robbi was asked to write an article against homoeopathy which was meant to be its death-blow, but he declined from lack of time and recommended his young assistant, Dr Hering, to undertake the work. Hering was pleased to be asked to do this and set about to read as much as possible of Hahnemann's writings. Finding much that was new to him, he determined to investigate these propositions thoroughly in order to refute more positively the points that Hahnemann had set before the profession. Calling on an apothecary in Leipzig whom he knew, Hering asked for some *Cinchona* and was asked, 'What do you want it for?' To which he replied, 'For the purpose of proving it in order the more thoroughly to attack the new folly.' To this the druggist said, 'Let it alone, Hering, you are treading on dangerous ground.' Hering answered that he did not fear the truth. The article was not written; for Hering was to become an able champion of homoeopathy.

While still a medical student, as he was dissecting, Hering received a wound which did not respond to treatment. His hand became so inflamed and infected that amputation was advised. A friend of his, who was a student of Hahnemann's, suggested trying a potentized drug. This resulted in a complete cure and was the means of thoroughly converting Hering to the value of homoeopathy. Indeed, so thoroughly was Hering convinced that the law of cure had been discovered that he wrote his marginal thesis on '*De Medicina Futura*' which was a forcible defence of the law of cure. He then publicly announced his conversion to homoeopathy without reservation to Robbi and his publisher. It was then considered probable that his upholding of the homoeopathic 'heresy' might prejudice him in the eyes of the Leipzig professors and he was advised to take his degree at Würzburg, where he graduated in 1826. He was then appointed house-physician in the Dresden Hospital.

Soon after he was qualified he was appointed by the King of Saxony to accompany the Saxon legation to Dutch Guiana in order to do scientific research and prepare zoological collections for the government. He and his wife, therefore, left for Surinam with another scientist. He maintained his post for several years, but during the course of time he was more and more drawn into the practice of medicine on Hahnemannian principles. Here he met with great success which was capped when he cured the Governor's daughter of what was thought a fatal disease.

While in Dutch Guiana collecting botanical and geological specimens, he was alone, except for his wife, with the native Indians. They had told him so much about the Surukuku snake, their name for the bushmaster (*Lachesis muta*), and its powerful venom that he offered a reward for a live specimen. When they finally captured one and presented it to Hering, in a box, directly he set it down to open the case they fled. Carefully holding the snake's head, Hering 'milked' the venom onto granules of sugar of milk. In his description of his experiment Hering said that the mere handling of the poison and working with it in its first stages of dilution was enough to 'throw him into a high fever with delirium and mania'. At last he slept. On waking his first questions were, 'What did I do? What did I say?' His wife remembered well enough and the symptoms were carefully recorded. That was the first proving of *Lachesis* which over the years has saved many lives.

It is interesting that Hering could never tolerate tight clothing around his neck, and during the proving of *Lachesis* this symptom annoyed him more than usual. This special symptom has been confirmed many times in practice since then, both as a local symptom of the neck and as a dislike of tight clothing on the body generally.

During his residence in Surinam he continued his occasional contributions to the *Homoeopathic Archives* which he had first done in 1825. The King of Saxony was prevailed upon by his court physician and a directive was sent to Hering to attend to his duties as a collector and let medical matters alone. Hering resented such intolerance and promptly resigned his appointment.

Not long after he gave up his position with the King of Saxony he took up practice in Paramaribo. But this did not last very long.

Hering's friend and former pupil, Dr George Bute induced him to go to America and work in homoeopathy there. He went to Philadelphia very early in 1833, stayed a short while and then had a bit of bad luck elsewhere before setting up again in Philadelphia, this time permanently. As early as 1834 he said, 'I told my pupils: in studying disease think that all remedies may help in a case; in studying a remedy think that it may help in every disease.'

In spite of his very large practice he found time to write much and to superintend the work of many young and less experienced men. His Saturday night meetings attended by students and young practitioners were praised as a boon.

Hering was the first one to carry out provings on a snake venom but was also the first to suggest the use of nosodes— a remedy extracted from the product of a specific disease made up in minute substances to cure that same disease— for what might be termed an oral vaccine. In 1831 he suggested the prevention and cure of hydrophobia and smallpox by the proving of their poisons. In 1833 he introduced *Lyssin*, prepared from the saliva of a mad dog as a cure for hydrophobia more than half a century before Pasteur proclaimed his discovery. Also in 1831, in Europe, Hahnemann published his provings of *Psorinum*, his first nosode prepared from 'itch', in the *Homoeopathic Journal*.

Weber, also in Europe, had read Hering's suggestions and made a preparation of *Anthracinum* from the spleen of animals affected by anthrax. In 1838 in Leipzig he published a treatise about an epidemic of anthrax treated successfully with *Anthracinum* in which he claims he cured every case in both animals and men. It was not until 1876 and 1883 that Robert Koch published his findings in the treatment of this disease.

Working in Philadelphia Hering did not forget his friends in Dutch Guiana and in 1835 he published the *Homoeopathic Domestic Physician* expressly for the missionaries in the colony. The book was so popular that it went into 29 editions in English and German and was translated into French, Spanish, Italian, Danish, Hungarian, Russian and Swedish.

Working with Dr Wesselhoeft Hering founded the North American Academy of the Homoeopathic Healing Art; it was the first homoeopathic institute in the world. After Hahnemann's death in Paris his widow tried to persuade Hering to join her, but he declined. Instead in the next few years he and his colleagues in Philadelphia originated and founded the American Institute of Homoeopathy, the American Provers's Union, the Homoeopathic Medical College and the Hahnemann Medical College of Philadelphia. It was there he held the chair of Institutes and Materia Medica from 1867 until his death thirteen years later. Between the years 1850 and 1860 four more colleges of homoeopathic medicine were organized in the United States of America; in Cleveland in 1850, St Louis in 1857, Chicago in 1859 and New York, finally in 1860.

Hering's energy was astonishing. Beside teaching, organizing, and administering, he was interested in methodical provings. In 1850 he introduced the North American witch hazel, *Hamamelis virginiana* to the pharmacopoeia. Dr Tyler wrote of him, 'At the beginning of his teaching career at Allentown he lectured and published in German, which had Hahnemann's approval, and he wrote to Hering in 1836 telling him that he need not be afraid of English competition as there was so far no English translation of the most important homoeopathic works.'

In 1867, on behalf of the Hahnemann Medical College of Philadelphia, Hering asked Hahnemann's widow's permission to translate the sixth edition of the *Organon* which, although completed in 1842, was still in manuscript form. Madame Hahnemann refused. Hering's own monumental work, *Guiding Symptoms*, based on fifty years of clinical practice began to appear in 1879. In the preface of the first volume he wrote, 'It has been my rule through life never to accept anything as true unless it came as near mathematical proof as possible in its domain of science. On the other hand I never reject anything as false unless there was stronger proof of its falsity.'

He died suddenly, 23 July 1880.

4

Homoeopathy in Practice

I want at this point to give illustrations of the application of homoeopathy. This book is not meant to be a *Materia Medica*. Those are already written by Kent, Clarke, Richard Hughes, Allen, Tyler and others. Although some are put in rather old-fashioned language, the picture of the remedies cannot be bettered. Homoeopathy is not a philosophy, it is a science based on observation and experience. The homoeopath keeps to a principle, and has done so scientifically for at least the past 170 years because the principle does not change. Fashion in ordinary medicine tends to alter quickly with the announcement of each new refinement of technique. Looking back over the centuries doctors tried bleeding, purging and blunderous prescribing. When these methods were proved inefficient, and surgical techniques became safer from the nineteenth century onwards, teeth and tonsils were extracted for all manner of medical ills. This was succeeded by the widespread application of the Sulpha drugs, this in turn was followed by the antibiotics to which germs quickly became resistant, or to which the patient developed a sensitivity. Cortisone was the rage until the discovery of the devastating side-effects restricted its use. And now there is a different tranquillizer to be prescribed for any variety of stress ailments; and these may be given without knowing which is best suited to the patient. But the homoeopathic doctor, because he knows his patient knows how to fit his drug to the individual.

Whooping cough still occurs in spite of inoculations, and I remember being called to see a delicate child of seven, who, though she did not whoop, had such a distressing cough I thought this was whooping cough, somewhat masked by her former inoculation. I gave her homoeopathic *Drosera*. She progressed rapidly, and in a short time was free from any cough. The local doctor, who had asked me to see the child, asked the mother if there was any way of getting this medicine, as his own children had kept him and his wife awake for five weeks. I sent him some *Drosera*, and the children had lost their coughs in a week.

Pulsatilla is often found useful in treating certain types of people in the first spell of hot weather. Children who need this remedy wilt in the heat and are most frequently fair-haired, plump and rosy cheeked. They are often described as 'sensitive' and demand attention. They are apt to be headachy, particularly after eating too much fat or rich food. They are prone to rubbing their eyes which have been irritated by the wind. There is also an extra tendency for styes to form on the upper lids. These patients needing *Pulsatilla* usually get a lot of catarrh with sneezing, and the nasal discharge can be yellow and offensive. Furthermore they often get a tickling-scraping cough and if they get a cold it is worse in the evening. On lying down they feel forced to sit up to get rid of the yellow mucus which accumulates. If toothache occurs it is worse for a warm drink. They crave cold water to wash their mouths and feel much better when cold air blows on them. Their pharynx can be very dry in the morning. There is usually a definite desire for food, appetite is characterized by a distinct liking for sweet things and *no thirst*. The patients are subject to a variety of gurglings and nausea or even pain in the stomach an hour or two after food. *Pulsatilla* is one of the best remedies for enuresis. On the whole these patients are poor sleepers. They cannot get off because of something on their minds, especially after eating too much and too late. A strong characteristic is that they sleep with their arms above their heads. *Pulsatilla* is a great rheumatic remedy, particularly for a single joint, like a knee. But it is also effective for wandering rheumatism which attacks first one joint and then another, usually worse in the summer and aggravated by heat.

A boy of eight was taken to the Homoeopathic Hospital's out-patients department. His mother described him as cheerful and very good temperamentally. She said he wept very easily but never got angry, in spite of having a rather domineering and bad-tempered sister of ten. The boy could never eat fat, or rich food, but he liked cakes and sweets, almost abnormally. He could not stand hot weather. When he was a baby, he was never able to be left in his pram in the sun. He was not ill, but had no energy and wilted in the heat. Even then, with the summer over, he could not seem to pick up. With such a definite history he was given *Pulsatilla*. The next month, when he returned, he looked very much better and stood up as if he had enough energy to meet anything.

The mother was very pleased, but she was even happier about her daughter. Because this cross, irritable little girl, whose extreme irritability caused reactions every day in the family, was quite a different child to live with after having *Nux vomica*.

When the homoeopathic doctor is prescribing for patients he tries to find out what is called the constitutional remedy.

The mother of a ten-year-old girl took her daughter to a homoeopathic doctor for treatment. In her youth her own mother, now long dead, had treated all the family with homoeopathic medicine. Now the anxious mother of the ten-year-old longed to try the treatment that her own mother had so believed in. The girl was a plump, stocky little child, very pale, but quite capable of giving her own symptoms. She gave her history and then produced a book which carefully listed the times of her bowel actions, both night and day. This revealed that she had had ten to fifteen bowel actions in twenty-four hours (day and night), and that sometimes there was a lot of blood. When asked about her appetite, she looked hurriedly at her mother, and then admitted that she liked eating *soap*. The doctor then learned that her bag and all her pockets were filled with thin slivers of soap; her mother went on to say that they were found in her satchel, schoolbooks and even in her hymn-book. Her marked desire for soap was even more extreme when her colitis (ulcerated large bowel) was aggravated. Also the little girl had a great tendency to worry and was extremely sensitive to any criticism. At night she sweated profusely around the head, although she was generally a chilly child. She had been very slow in learning to walk and in getting her first teeth. Only recently had she been able to keep up with the other children at school. She was so pale that she was admitted to hospital at once. It was found that her haemoglobin level was only 40% and she was given a blood transfusion. Soon after she was given *Calcarea carbonica* 10 m and this was not repeated for a year. Her health improved steadily and satisfactorily. The pediatrician who had seen her when she was six thought then that she most certainly at some time would require surgery for her bowel condition, but now found at a later date that she was doing very well. He asked to see her four years later and if possible when she was seventeen. At the time of the last visit he said he was very pleased and that she was quite well, and that there was no question of the need for an operation. The same pediatrician wrote to the homoeopathic doctor a few years later asking if he would like to have a further shot at another extremely interesting, but very difficult case.

In this particular instance the case which the pediatrician wanted the homoeopathic doctor to see concerned a twenty-month old child. The little girl was suffering from a case of *Osteogenesis imperfecta*, a little understood disease. She was unable to sit or stand because her bones were too weak, and had to be strapped onto a tray which had been made for her. A hole in the tray gave her space through which she could move one arm, and there she stayed all day. In spite of everything she was a cheerful little child. She was very pale, but ate well. However if she were left alone near the coal-box, she was inclined to reach out and eat a piece of coke or a cinder. Her feet and hands were very cold and damp. During the night she sweated very profusely around the head. Sometimes she woke screaming from night terrors. The doctor gave her a high potency of *Calcarea carbonica* and said he would see her again in three months. When he arrived the second time, she was sitting on the edge of the sofa waiting to show him how she could get round the room holding on to the furniture. She was seen by the homoeopathic doctor every three months for the next three years until the family had to move because the father had obtained a better job. On the last visit when the doctor arrived a little figure was waiting at the top of a slope ready to ride down on her tricycle to greet him. The mother has written several times to report on the progress of her daughter. She attends an ordinary school and keeps up well with the other children. She plays games and the only defect she has is a slight curvature.

Let me go on to give one or two examples of constitutional prescribing: nearly twenty years ago, a homoeopathic doctor was visited by a woman of seventy. She was a renowned gardener, but now found that her work was getting difficult. She was full of aches and pains, and all this was much worse for the cold. On shaking hands with her, the doctor noticed how dry and cold her hands were. She was a thin, pale, anxious individual with very quick movements. She walked very rapidly into the doctor's consulting room, glanced around quickly and started to recite her history before she sat down. She looked alive and the only calm thing about her was her expression. She was very much 'on the spot'. She first mentioned her rheumatism, but had much more to tell. At her age, she felt, it was pretty hopeless; no one could do anything for her. Then she gave her real story. She had a lot of discomfort in her stomach. It was much worse when she bent, and when it became too much to bear she had to go in and lie down in the midst of her gardening activities. She was sure in her mind that this was 'the beginning of the end', and something very serious, and she thought no one could help her. She had always had a small appetite. But, the food had to be perfectly fresh and it upset her if it were not. Another thing was that the very smell of food would sometimes make her feel sick. When the pain in her stomach was bad, she felt 'off her food' except for milk, possibly coffee or something sour. But she had to be careful. Fruit might cause diarrhoea. If she were thirsty she liked something by her to sip—she never drank it down at once. When her stomach was painful vegetables, iced food or even alcohol could upset her. Next, she admitted to the doctor, she was a real fusser and over-anxious about everything. When her grandson was late getting back at weekends she got into a panic. If she had a dinner party her cook, whom she had had for years, would almost give notice because she went into the kitchen eight or ten times to remind her of something, or to see that an item of food was not put on to cook too soon. After losing her husband and three sons during the war she was never without a night light in her bedroom. She looked after the place for her grandson, and was always afraid that something would go wrong, not with herself so much as with her family. She was full of apprehension and in an acute state of stress which made her feel almost suicidal. Whilst recounting her history she was very restless and constantly on the move, opening and shutting her bag or waving her foot up and down.

Later she was X-rayed and found to have a hiatus hernia but nothing else seriously wrong. She was given a high potency of *Arsenicum album* and asked to write to the doctor and report after a month. She did not do this and the doctor wondered how she had fared. Then at the end of nine months she sent a letter to say 'I really think I am better for the medicine I have been given, but I am too old and too far gone to benefit further! However, I will be coming up to London anyway and wonder if I could be seen again to have another try?' The doctor saw her and gave her another dose of *Arsenicum album* with equally good results. She still does her gardening, opening it to the public and organizes things very well. She lives a happy and useful life and today is nearly ninety. She has taken her constitutional remedy every few months over the past twenty years. Much of her good health is due to her strong constitution and to the stabilizing effect of the homoeopathic remedy.

We have found three highly successful methods of treating hay-fever homoeopathically. The first is by giving a patient his constitutional remedy. In 1964, a boy was seen with very troublesome hay-fever. It started in May or even during a warm April and lasted until the middle of July.

He was then sixteen years old and had been troubled since he was eight. He had had injections against it for two years running, but they had not helped. The patient was tall, thin and delicate looking with fair hair. He was narrow chested and inclined to stoop and seemed anaemic; he was obviously bright and intelligent. In talking to the doctor he hardly took his eyes off him and appeared as if he were longing for reassurance. He told the doctor that he could play games and do anything. The outstanding feature of a patient responding to *Phosphorus* is hypersensitivity; and this boy showed it at once in his history. He was very impressionable to his surroundings and could be wildly enthusiastic about some idea. Yet he described himself as being rather disinclined to exert himself in general. His most prominent emotion was fear. He was afraid of being alone, of the dark, of thunder, or of what might happen, of being ill. He felt particularly unwell when it was twilight. He had quite a good appetite, but was easily upset by hot food and drink. He much preferred his food cold especially if he had an upset stomach. Yet after having swallowed it and it became warm in his stomach he often vomited. He had a great desire for salt. He was a very chilly boy. He was apt to get a night hunger and had to have something to eat before going to bed. He was a perfect picture of one who responds to *Phosphorus*. He has needed a repeat once or twice, but now considers that he is free from hay-fever.

The second method of using homoeopathy in hay-fever is by finding a remedy that covers the general symptoms. *Sabadilla* is a remedy that has been used for many years. The patient comes for his hay-fever and describes his frequent running nose (coryza) and violent spasmodic sneezing accompanied by watering eyes and a bewildered feeling in the head. He often complains of feeling as if there were a soft lump in the throat which he has to swallow. This he says comes on with a marked regularity but the sneezing fits are more or less continual. This type of hay-fever may come early in the season. The patient is very chilly and shivery and particularly dislikes cold food and drink but is helped by hot food and drink.

Twenty-one years ago when he was thirty-five, Major S went for treatment to help his acute catarrh in the hay-fever season. This usually began with a rawness in the nose and severe bouts of sneezing. The discharge became thicker and thicker and he could not breathe through his nose. He was always much better if he could inhale hot air and would be found in the airing cupboard with the heater full on, or lighting a fire and kneeling in front of it on quite a mild day. He was also very sensitive to the smell of certain flowers; if in England he got 'Rose fever' or later on hay-fever from newly mown grass. These were often accompanied by an unpleasant sore throat beginning on the left and spreading to the right side and again relieved by inhaling hot air. He was given *Sabadilla* for four years after which he considered himself cured. Then after fifteen years he returned because of a sudden and acute recurrence of his symptoms. The *Sabadilla* was repeated and he was again, and remains, free of attacks.

Euphrasia officinalis (eye-bright) was used as an eye medicine by the ancients and homoeopathic experiments have fully confirmed its old time reputation. Some patients have a sensation of dust or sand in the eyes and *Euphrasia* is extremely useful in some cases of hay-fever accompanied by lachrymation and sneezing. It is also useful as an eye lotion in a mixture of five drops in an eye-glass of water. There was an amusing incident which a patient told in the course of giving her history. She was having great trouble with sneezing, a running nose and severely watering eyes. Her eye specialist had been giving her cortisone eye drops to relieve the condition. After visiting her ophthalmic surgeon she went into a restaurant for a cup of coffee and a man suddenly leaned over the table and said to her 'You must have help for your eyes. Do go to the Homoeopathic pharmacy and get *Euphrasia* eye-drops.' As she felt desperate she did this and found great relief. When she next went for an eye check-up the consultant asked her 'Have you been doing anything different for your eyes? They are so definitely better.' She told him about the *Euphrasia* and had to sit quietly while he looked it up in various *Materia Medica* to see if he could find anything about it. He could not at that moment, but he recommended her to go on with it and said he would make further enquiries.

The third method of treating hay-fever is by using potencies of the particular flower or substance to which the patient is sensitive. There are many whose attacks start when coming near newly mown grass because they are sensitive to Timothy grass. *Phleum pratense* is the medicine made from this and many patients are quickly relieved by the 12th potency. If the attacks start a little later these are usually due to some pollen to which the person is particularly sensitive. A homoeopathic preparation of mixed pollens 30 taken for two or three weeks will often control the trouble. Finally there is a group of patients who are very sensitive to the moulds from trees, particularly in the late summer and early autumn, and these respond well to M. A. P. (*Mucor, Aspergillus* and *Penicillium*).

An elderly woman worried all her friends and family by having a very troublesome deep cough. When asked about it she explained that she had always been prone to hay-fever and of recent years this cough was its present manifestation. She had very little sneezing, no one was to worry as the cough would clear in the winter. On that history she was given homoeopathic M.A.P. and to her surprise the cough had gone in about ten days.

In writing about homoeopathy one must also mention the neurotic patient who is given tranquillizers, probably sleeping pills and sometimes even anti-depressants for treatment. As a rule these patients have no actual disease, and are not really ill, but they find it very difficult to live a normal life and are often afraid of tackling a job. They come to the doctor with a great many symptoms which they like to describe fully but which quite often mean very little. It is not at all easy to deal with them, but through the years patients have been given their constitutional remedy and it has helped considerably. In these cases one likes to use a high potency and see how much it will do but there are often so many complaints that it is justifiable to give a low potency of a remedy like *Coffea* or *Lycopodium* to help the sleepless, or *Argentum nitricum* to the patient who dares not go shopping alone or who may become panicky if she feels closed in. *Aurum* 6 can be useful if they are depressed and down in health at the same time, or they may be greatly helped by *Natrum mur* 6 if they feel rather resentful that life has not treated them better. It is very gratifying to find them once again taking on responsibilities whether at home or at work.

In concluding this chapter I want to show what the homoeopathic remedy can do in an acute condition. The common cold takes many forms, but most of us have experienced it. In each susceptible person it seems to run to type. In the last twenty years scientists have isolated innumerable viruses which are associated with various forms of catarrhal conditions. We homoeopaths might well say that today there may be as many viruses but there have always been remedies to cope with the individual who experiences the cold syndrome.

Let me illustrate what I mean, first of all with *Aconite*. The type of cold best treated with this remedy has a sudden onset after exposure to cold dry winds. The cold will start a few hours after exposure, with a dry, stinging sensation in the nose. There will be a rapid rise in temperature, a roaring in the ears accompanied by sleeplessness. There is sneezing, and a hot fluid coryza; the throat feels as if it is burning, and the larynx is sensitive to touch externally. There is an anxious restlessness and fearfulness, and all these symptoms are aggravated at night. If *Aconite* is taken frequently at the beginning, the cold will clear up in twenty four hours.

Now an acute cold may occur in a patient with an *Arsenicum* constitution as I have described it in the case of the seventy-year-old lady who loved gardening, but it may affect anyone. It has certain characteristics which mark it out from all the rest; the type of discharge is one of them. There is a watery pouring from the nose that excoriates the upper lip. The patient is liable to take cold at changes of weather, and sneezes a great deal at the beginning, because of an irritable spot in the front of the nose. If the cold is not checked it may quickly go onto the chest. The patient feels very chilly, and may complain that there is ice cold blood flowing through his vessels. Any aches or pains he may have are burning, he loves to hug the fire and is always better for heat. He may wake up at one o'clock in the morning with a wheezing sort of a cough, without any expectoration. He will be restless, and anxious, but is much chillier than the *Aconite* patient.

Nux vomica is needed when a cold starts with one very irritating, raw spot high up in the back of the nostril. The patient cannot move without feeling chilly. A teasing cough may develop which is painful and spasmodic, and he may feel sick with it. There may be pain in the larynx and a feeling that something is torn loose in the chest when coughing. I heard of a homoeopathic doctor giving it to one of his patients who having just returned from a business trip abroad found himself surrounded by lots of colds. He told his doctor: 'I've just the feeling in my nose that I am going to get a cold, and I must have something to stop it, because of all the reports I have to give.' He was given *Nux vomica* 10 m and sneezed his head off all night long, but felt perfectly well the next day. He is never without his bottle of *Nux vomica* and will take it to stop his colds developing.

Causticum is another remedy for the common cold with quite a different picture. It starts with dryness in the back of the throat and a feeling of rawness extending downwards. There is often a dry tickling cough with only a little expectoration after a long paroxysm of coughing. Mucus collects in the back of the throat, and the sufferer feels exceedingly uncomfortable and may make an awful noise in trying to dislodge it and often will finally have to swallow it. The eyes water terribly on going into the open air, and there is a lot of blinking. These patients very often have a heaviness of the upper eyelid with a cold, and this gives them one of the general causticum symptoms; a weakness of the muscles and thus a tendency for the eyes to close. It may be one sided. There is also a lot of morning sneezing and a blockage of the nostrils. There is often a frequency of urination with the colds, sometimes incontinence on sneezing or coughing or blowing the nose. There may be a hoarseness and loss of voice or difficulty speaking.

Hepar sulph. is another remedy one thinks of in cold dry weather. It can be useful when there is a sticking sensation in the back of the throat, like a splinter, and there may be paroxysms of dry teasing cough at the beginning of a cold. The chest will be sore, and the patient will want to keep covered up; the cough may come on from any draught that creeps under the bed-clothes. The patient is chilly, but sweats a lot without relief. He is very irritable and is apt to quarrel with his own shadow if there is nothing else to quarrel with. There is a suffocative croupy cough in the middle of the night, but *Hepar sulph.* given early will stop a bronchitis developing. This frequently is a remedy for those types of influenza whose symptoms match these.

Ferrum phosph. can be prescribed when the cold develops into a pleural involvement quickly. It starts with a sharp stabbing pain in the chest, with muscular soreness of the chest wall which is worse on motion. There is a dislike of talking, and the patient wants to lie quite silent and is terribly sensitive to noise. He has an abnormal thirst for large quantities of cold liquid of some kind, and has a singularly uncoated tongue. The tongue may be red, darkish and inflamed looking. These patients have the most tormenting, persistent, irritating cough, with intense soreness in the chest, and if you percuss their chests, they do not like it at all, as it is apt to be painful.

The last two remedies I want to tell you about I used to call my Number 1 and Number 2 cold pills. I do not find the need for them so often indicated today because of the changing pattern of infection which has come in the wake of the wide use of antibiotics. There used to be a lot of bacterial infection associated with colds, but the anti-biotics have killed off the common streptococci and staphylococci and pneumococci, and allowed the viruses to take over, so I don't find *Gelsemium* and *Bryonia* quite so commonly needed. But because of this change I think I ought to mention them.

As in conventional medicine, so in homoeopathy it is essential that the patient does not continue for too long on any medicine. An extended overdosage of any medicine, no matter how beneficial, invariably causes damage.

In practice homoeopathy has never isolated itself from investigating new scientific and medicinal techniques Nor will it refrain from employing allopathic medicines as a temporary measure in an emergency, especially in cases of dramatic upset to the heart or endocrinal system. But once the crisis has been passed successfully, continued homoeo-pathic treatment will often complete the cure.

5

Taking the Case

Homoeopathy is a system of medicine practised by men and women within the body of the medical profession. We have all taken our orthodox medical degrees. All doctors diagnose along the same lines. We all use pathological tests, blood tests, X-ray analyses—every form of investigation that may be necessary is common to every branch of practising medicine. As I have already mentioned, the homoeopathic doctor tries to find the totality of the symptoms of the patient. I would emphasize that it is on the patient's reaction to stress that the homoeopathic doctor prescribes, and that no physical aspect or response to treatment is unimportant. Ever since psychosomatic medicine was first thought of, more and more has been talked and written about stress; but apart from psychology, the use of vaccines and antiallergents, little difference is made in the actual treatment; but to the homoeopathic doctor it is the patient's reaction to stress that is all important. It is well for those interested in homoeopathy to be reminded that we are not fighting a disease as such, but are helping a patient in his reaction to stress, whether it be mental, emotional, physical, bacterial or just because the everyday stress and strain of life has become too much. It is an enthralling study and one gets to recognize the symptomatic pattern given by the patient which then suggests so many remedies.

Ever since I started in practice I have had open consultations one morning a week, and patients arrive without an appointment for homoeopathic treatment from anywhere in the country or from abroad. The number of visitors to the clinic varies; some days there may be only ten, on another there may be forty. Whatever the number I always make a point of fetching each patient from the waiting room, and it is astonishing what one can learn just while leading them to the consulting room.

Upon entering the waiting room it is essential to notice every detail about the patient. For what we see and note can so often be something of which the patient himself may be unaware, or, in some cases, may be something which he thinks he has concealed. There are some who are obvious immediately; such as the woman who was so terrified of draughts that she kept an open umbrella over her head.

One notices the young adult sitting opposite the door who is patently very tense—that sullen, resentful expression surely means he has been forced to see a doctor. The two women sitting together in very friendly, bright conversation, both pleased to meet again and enjoying themselves mightily. The teenage boy who has produced a book from his pocket and is busy reading it, to the utter exclusion of a boy his own age seated next to him. This lad has a frown, and looks worried; this and his rather detached attitude, make one feel quite certain that after hearing his case history *Lycopodium* will be prescribed. Without their saying a word the patients can tell so much to the experienced homoeopathic doctor. We already know much about the teenager who does not take his eyes off you, who badly needs reassurance, and yet seems bright and intelligent, who so often has a glint in the hair. One notices if the patient is well-groomed or untidy. Then again, the appearance of the skin and hair helps the homoeopathic doctor in his diagnosis: a blotchy complexion, a tendency to skin eruptions, acne; cracks in the corners of the mouth, or on the lips; whether the hair is fine, coarse or greasy; horny finger nails, cracked fingertips; crusted eyelashes; or even the slightly blue tinge in the eyeballs. We also gain information from the way the patient gets up and walks in. The deliberate stride of the man who has come to give his history, who wants to give it and get it over, who may be rather flushed on first arriving, puts his brief case down, but does it with a slight tremor. This man may suddenly turn sallow, or perhaps greasy immediately after entering the consulting room. Sometimes he does have poor skin, or he might have a rash at his hairline. He is the one who needs *Natrum muriaticum*. Or the neat elderly patients who are very nervous, very restless and who enter the room quickly, glance alertly round them, and begin their histories before there is time to write down their names and addresses. All these traits suggest a treatment of *Arsenicum*.

Just from shaking hands with a patient one can learn a lot. One notices the cold, dry hand typical of the person who responds successfully to *Arsenicum*; or the cold, damp hand which may suggest *Hepar sulph.*; be the hand rough and cracked with overgrown nails and *Silica* comes to mind; is the hand cold, damp, limp to the point of seeming boneless?—*Calcarea carbonica* is what is needed; then the firm handshake, particularly firm if he is grateful for improved health resulting from a treatment with *Lycopodium*. Is there profuse sweating of the hands? There was that nineteen-year-old girl whose hands dripped with sweat. She was working for what she called 'a high-power' boss, and she had to redo most of her typing because the paper got so wet and smeared. She also had to wear a jackinette apron under the back of her skirt, she sweated so badly that it soaked through; she was cured by *Thuja*.

But we must always remember that no single condition suggests the remedy; it is not only the general appearance, nor the single factor of the condition of the hair, the complexion, the stride or the handshake, but the combination of factors that lead the homoeopathic doctor to prescribe for the particular patient.

By looking at children as you get to know them you will learn through experience how to classify them. The untidy child who looks as if his clothes were dragged on, with very red mucous membranes lining his eyes, very red, nearly raw, lips, who is rather dirty and hates a bath; the child who is often very hungry and loves to eat fat. I remember a man asking me if anything could be done for his grandson, who was just that sort of boy—he always looked so scruffy. We were at a garden party. The grandfather and friends were standing near a big table set out with chocolate biscuits, cream buns, scones, jam and everything that any seven-year-old would crave. The boy approached the table, and after looking at it very carefully, stretched out his hand, and drew a dish of butter pats towards him and proceeded to eat every one! These children are characteristically those whose health improves when given *Sulphur*.

Or the bright, intelligent, eager child who sometimes perspires leaving beads of sweat on the upper lip and forehead because of nervousness at coming to a doctor, but who, otherwise, never perspires without reason. Who, again, keeps his eye on you all the time until his turn comes, and who badly needs reassurance. The mother will most likely tell us that when the child is unwell he cannot lie on his left side, and that his most comfortable position is lying propped up with his head back. He most likely needs *Phosphorus*.

Silica is for the child who comes in nervously, or is dragged in by his mother. He is generally listless and uninterested, but not frightened; he just feels and looks poorly. When in good form he is delightful and friendly, but should he be mismanaged or unwell he can look belligerent and stolid. Sometimes it is better to see him on his own. He has a pale, sickly face, with an eruption around the eyes, rough, yellow nails and very cold feet, probably damp to the touch and frequently offensive to smell. He sits hunched up as if huddled against a chill, and yet starts to sweat, particularly around the head. Most prevalent, and a decisive factor in prescribing *Silica*, is a tendency towards skin eruptions on the chin, neck and elsewhere.

When we are asked to see as a patient a child who is fat, fair, flabby and very pale, who is often dumped into a chair, and sits there smiling round at everyone, not stirring and sweating quite profusely in a cool room, whose general aspect is one of being heavy and weak, then we feel that *Calcarea carbonica* will very likely greatly improve the condition. This is especially so when the parent tells us that at night the child's pillow is soaked, he perspires so much. As he gets older we find he usually becomes a worrier, and is apt to suffer from night-terrors. At school this type gets a reputation for being slow; he cannot keep up with others of his own age, either in work or games, this frequently bothers him, for he is aware of his short comings and makes him very sensitive to criticism.

Psorinum works wonders on patients who so often are greasy and dusky, of an unwashed, dirty appearance, whose thin limbs are covered with a harsh, dry skin; who are described in some books as the 'unwashable'. *Psorinum*, incidentally, is one of the rare remedies for certain asthmatic children: the type who, in trying to ease their breathing, lie flat on their backs with their arms stretched out. This patient very much resembles in his characteristics those who respond well to *Sulphur*, but is unlike them in one aspect; they suffer intensely from the cold.

A patient's skin condition reveals much, as we have stated, and someone with glowing red cheeks and dry, burning skin among his other symptoms is often best treated with *Belladonna*. This is very useful when administered early on when they are acutely flushed and the skin is hot, red, dry, with throbbing sensations which are burning to the touch. The patient twitches in his sleep and often when ill enough to be delirious, has to be held down, and spits at everyone around him.

A frequent patient among the young with the physical characteristics of being, again, fair-skinned, blonde, blue-eyed, and, on the whole, plump and engaging, but who also likes fuss and being petted, for some reason will come into the consulting room tearful and hiding behind her mother, and yet for no reason, will then be laughing. This very changeable child may often go faint in a hot room, they certainly wilt in the first heat of summer. They are thirstless children, who hate fat, and like sweet things. Their eyes are often strained or weakened, making them subject to styes, and at night will sleep with their arms above their heads. We treat these children with their fluctuating temperaments and physiques with *Pulsatilla*, which comes from the *Pulsatilla vulgaris* 'the wind flower': the remedy, like the patient is very changeable, and is often referred to as the 'weather-cock remedy'.

Chamomilla, on the other hand, is known as the 'can't bear it' remedy, and we prescribe it for sick children who are in a turmoil in their tempers: the infant who whines and howls and insists on being carried about. The moment father puts his baby down, the child begins again; he holds out his hands for things and no sooner given them pushes them away in disgust. This calming drug brings peace to the household within minutes and more fathers have been converted to homoeopathy by the use of this remedy than by any other drug.

Once in the consulting room it is essential to record the case history carefully and to pay strict attention to what the patient has to say and to let him tell his story in his own way. How many of our patients tell us 'It is so nice to have someone who will sit and listen to me.' Friends and relations who accompany the patient may have points to add to his history. Once he has told of his complaint it is necessary to enquire into his family history, his own past history— which is often most important to the homoeopath—and any hereditary or latent diseases which may have occurred. There are many other things that the homoeopathic doctor will want to know in order to get a picture of the whole patient. One has to find out about the patient's appetite: is it good, and has it varied recently? Does any food upset him? does he dislike something particularly? has he a special craving for sweets? salt? spicy foods? meat fat? fish? eggs? milk? Is he thirsty? hot or cold drinks? and how much at a time? a full glass at one go? or just to sip? Does he prefer hot or cold food? is he ever dyspeptic or flatulent after eating? or at any time of day? or particular hour?

Then there is sleep. Does the patient go to sleep quickly, or is his brain so active that he goes on working out things and does not relax? How much does he dream? does he suffer from nightmares? occasionally or frequently? does he find himself awake and screaming? Is there any favourite position when sleeping? on his face? or with his arms above his head? on one side rather than the other?

When Hahnemann organized his provings and made

systematic the principles of homoeopathic medicine he emphasized over and over again that the doctor must be particularly attentive to those symptons that are peculiar to the patient and characteristic of the patient, and not to be obsessed with the symptoms and characteristics that are common to the disease. After many years of experience Dr Kent stated that he regarded this advice of Hahnemann's to be the most vital point in the practice of homoeopathic medicine.

As a rule there is not much difficulty in recognizing the symptoms that are peculiar to the patient suffering from an acute disease. These usually appear in an ordinary manner and the common or pathological ones are well known. However, in chronic diseases this is not so easy, and it may be very difficult to separate the symptoms peculiar to the patient from those that are common to the disease. In long standing chronic cases the peculiar and characteristic symptoms may sometimes completely disappear or may have been utterly forgotten and so make our work of diagnosis that much more difficult. Naturally, in analyzing the symptoms which are specifically those of the patient as opposed to those which are common to the disease one has to be fully conversant with the latter. For instance: many serious kidney troubles have signs and symptoms in common; dysuria, oedema, palpitations and albuminuria; and we cannot determine the curative remedy from these alone. But if, in addition, the patient has a strong craving for fat, powerfully odoriferous urine and a chilling sensation in passing urine these indicate that *Nitric acid* is most likely the remedy.

There are various drugs that relieve the asthmatic, but again each case has to be considered on its own symptoms; we have earlier mentioned one in which *Psorinum* was most effective. But should the patient try to find relief in his breathing by lying on his face, or in the knee–elbow position this tells the homoeopathic doctor that *Medorrhinum* will bring relief. The observation that the patient does find comfort in this position is the essence of the difference of noting the symptoms typical of a disease, but prescribing for the individual who suffers from the disease. It must be remembered that all symptoms must be equally well marked, both in the patient and the remedy.

Once we have taken into account the symptoms that signify the patient, and those which identify the disease, we come upon another important division of symptoms: the distinction between the generals and the particulars. By the generals we mean those symptoms which affect the patient as a whole and are of the utmost importance in diagnosing for a remedy. The particulars are those symptoms that affect a specific organ. In treating the patient one must pay strict attention to what he may say of himself. Beside giving the details of what signify the infection he may be carrying he may give other bits of information such as saying 'I am thirsty.' 'I am cold.'. This shows that the whole of him is affected and not only one particular organ. A patient may have a number of gastric ailments combined with headaches, a roaring sensation in the ears, an aversion to fat and butter; all these tend to aggravate his condition. But if, in addition, the person is suffering from night-time diarrhoea, a nausea that arises after a hot, but not a cold, drink and has palpitations, these combined reactions strongly indicate the prescription of *Pulsatilla*. On the other hand, if there are a few strong general symptoms, such as an aversion to open air, and extreme susceptibility to cold in any form, then one would have to look to other remedies such as *Phosphorus* as these general symptoms are not those which respond readily to *Pulsatilla*, and we must find the medicine which best applies to the entire picture of the patient.

In taking a case Hahnemann said that the most important symptoms to search out are the mental ones, and it is the mental state which takes priority of consideration in the selection of the remedy. Yet it is the search for these symptoms which can be the most difficult task of all. For, so many patients are diffident about telling their inmost thoughts, nor do they like to reveal their yearnings and hatreds, their motives and fantasies, despite the fact that generally they are much relieved after doing so. There are so many mental states that consistently call for the same treatment because the symptoms are so consistent: those over fastidious patients, those whom we dub 'the man with the gold-headed cane' who so frequently respond marvellously to a course of *Arsenicum*; frequently the use of *Bryonia*, *Nux vomica* or *Chamomilla* calms those who suffer from extreme irritability; the gently lachrymose patient can become less tiresome after using *Pulsatilla*; and often the prescription of *Platina* changes a haughty personality to that of someone more affable and more approachable; then there are those who when ill become withdrawn, ungrateful and tyrannical and who have a complete *volte-face* when treated with *Phosphorus* or *Sepia*; many a would-be suicide after confessing to this deep distress, has taken on a new lease of life after taking *Cinchona* (quinine).

These in a way are simplifications, for mental states can vary in importance. The innermost workings of the mind are determined by attitudes of will and affection and these determine desires and aversions. One has to enquire after the prevailing moods, fluctuations of temper, what makes the patient angry, how he may react to grief or disappointment, what he fears, does he prefer solitude or company. Symptoms connected with intellect and memory are of some value, but less so than others. Sleep and dream patterns are of importance: those who suffer from a chronic grumpiness or aggravation upon awaking often need

Lachesis or *Sulphur*; the opposite temperament of those who are irritable due to loss of sleep benefit from *Cocculus* while a course of *Phosphorus* or *Sepia* will make others feel well with the world after a good sleep. Some people who are plagued with recurring dreams of throwing themselves from great heights are relieved of their painful nightmares after taking *Thuja*.

One invaluable general symptom is the effect of different temperatures. This will often help in deciding the remedy. But to be of use, the patient must be very definite in his reply to a question on how he is affected by heat or cold. He may state that he cannot stand heat; but it is not surprising on asking further questions to learn that what he really means is that he cannot abide a stuffy room and that he hates the cold. It is the definite answer to the definite question we need to help us in finding the remedy. Easy perspiration does not necessarily indicate that the patient suffers in hot weather; for those who respond to *Calcarea* are the very ones who are wont to sweat in a cold room and who by make-up generally feel very chilly. This question of temperature recurs in a patient whose whole body is markedly sensitive to a specific temperature and yet some specific part of him is sensitive to an opposite temperature. For instance: in acute illness some patients may feel extremely cold and yet are covered with cold sweat and find comfort in being fanned and will ask to have the window open in the coldest weather. We have found that *Carbo. vegetabilis* is the answer in these conditions, while on the other hand *Lycopodium* is most effective in curing those who are in discomfort when there is great heat and yet complain of stomach troubles and rheumatic pains, both of which should be improved when heat is applied. Then again, there are people who are only comfortable in what they describe as a medium temperature and who will suffer at either extreme of cold or heat. Many valuable hints are given when we are told of the effects that weather can have, hints that can indicate or reject a treatment. Take rheumatism; in many situations where we would expect the condition to be aggravated by a change in weather and yet find none, we then know that various drugs will prove ineffectual; so that if wet weather does not affect the rheumatism we can therefore eliminate *Calcarea*, *Rhus toxicodendron*, *Mercury*, *Natrum carbonicum*, *Natrum sulphuricum* and *Ruta*.

When trying to prescribe for the patient we must also take into consideration what reactions the patient may have to periods of, say, standing for a long while. Taking all things into account if there is unusual fatigue or aggravation to the system after standing which is peculiar to the patient then *Sulphur* might be indicated; whereas lying on the right side may further aggravate the symptoms and *Mercury* may be the remedy needed. Different sides of the body call for *Apis*, *Belladonna* and *Lycopodium* (if it is the right side) or we might consider *Argentum nitricum*, *Lachesis* or *Phosphorus* should the left side of the body be the site of the trouble.

Then again, we must consider how our diseases are influenced by time. We must recognize that it is not unusual for symptoms to become more aggravated at regular intervals. This can be a decisive factor in selecting the remedy. *Chelidonium*, *Natrum muriaticum* or *Nux vomica* are recommended when the suffering is most acute in the morning whereas evening recurrences of symptoms may indicate *Belladonna* or *Pulsatilla*. Some symptoms which only occur every other day make us look to *Cinchona*, *Sulphur* or *Lycopodium*; should the recurrence be, say, every two weeks, then we must consider *Arsenicum* or *Lachesis*. These last might apply equally well where the periodic return of symptoms is an uncommon occurrence in diseases. But this periodicity in individual patients usually signifies that special remedies are to be called for that have this same characteristic to a marked degree.

The cravings for, and aversions to, various food substances are general symptoms of importance. The aversion to fat is not uncommon to people who need *Pulsatilla*, and if by chance they eat fat it disagrees with them to a marked degree. An inordinate desire for salt could mean a prescription for *Natrum muriaticum* or *Phosphorus*, where we would give *Argentum nitricum* or *Lycopodium* to someone who constantly craves sweet things. These are a few examples of cravings which would indicate one remedy or another when the patient recognizes these hungers as having no physiological basis. In line with this there are the reactions to meals. Is there a feeling of discomfort in the stomach after eating, or relief? Does one feel the better or the worse for eating. And how significant are these reactions in prescribing treatment? We must take note especially when a patient is made better or worse in an area of the body having nothing to do with the stomach. If a pain elsewhere in the system should be relieved after a meal perhaps the patient requires *Natrum carbonicum* or *Kali bichromicum*. The effect of special foods on the entire system as well as on a specific portion of the body can be helpful. But, as a rule, only the digestive organs are affected and so these symptoms are only particulars. The special senses are indicative of the whole man, and give general symptoms as when he complains, for instance, that the odour of cooking food sickens him. But should he be offended by the smell of an open drain, or a disinfectant, this would be what we term a particular and as such is not as important a symptom. There is a very significant general which reveals itself in the blending of the generals and particulars into a harmonious whole. When all these characteristics fall into a specific and consistent pattern this condition assumes in our mind the name of the remedy for the disease. Thus those whose suffering in mind and body are so frequently cured by the wonderful drug *Sepia*, are called Sepia patients.

When the homoeopathic doctor talks of a Sepia type he has a specific picture in his mind. Every doctor remembers the tired looking, generally tall, thin, narrow-chested patient with the sallow complexion; the one whose face is sometimes discoloured by a saddle patch of yellow crossing the nose and running down the side of the face. Then the cheeks are often spotted with freckles or even brown patches; and although the face seems a bit fat for the figure it is frequently wrinkled and prematurely old-looking with a somewhat stupid expression.

Most Sepia types, strangely, are women; although this remedy can be needed by men. The woman patient often complains of a gnawing-empty feeling in the stomach; they are frequently constipated and have difficulty with bowel movements. They complain of a prolapse of the pelvic organs. She is many times to be discovered seated with one leg crossed over the other because only in this position does she feel comfortable. She is difficult in the home and tiresome to her neighbours. She is apt to lose affection for her husband and for her family. Envious of others who may have an easier life, she refuses offers of help in an insulting and peevish manner. My partner told me that it was after prescribing *Sepia* to a specific patient that she was convinced forever of the efficacy of homoeopathy. This is the story:

It happened when my partner was acting as a temporary substitute in another doctor's clinic. She was in the out-patients clinic of a homoeopathic hospital when she was noticed by a woman with her child who were on the point of leaving. Suddenly the woman stopped and approached my friend saying, 'Oh doctor! could you help me? I feel so awful and I can't go to a man doctor'. My partner was sympathetic and took her into a private dressing room and there took down the woman's history. She spoke of her tiredness and her dreads and of how bad tempered she was;

how she never had a smile for her husband when he came home. She felt that she had no love for him or her family. The world was black and she was afraid. After a moment the doctor left her for a bit. She then looked through the Repertory and finding what she sought prescribed *Sepia* 10m. and forgot all about her. Two months later walking through the out-patients department once again a woman rushed up, seized her hand and thanked her profusely. Her home and family life were restored to peace and happiness and her whole condition altered for the better. The change was so remarkable that it wasn't until my partner searched her records that she remembered the woman to whom she had given *Sepia* 10m.

There are two other points in homoeopathic case taking: one of these is the alternating of complaints, such as a stomach disorder being succeeded by eye trouble. Sometimes it is a mistake to treat the patient for the stomach and then to give him something to cure his eyes, because it is not infrequent that the constitutional remedy for this particular patient will cover all the symptoms displayed and will result in the cure of all his ailments. The other point to notice is the occurrence of a group of symptoms which we classify as 'strange, rare and peculiar'. An excellent example is found in the case of a patient with a temperature of 105° who nevertheless is absolutely thirstless; in which instance a treatment of *Pulsatilla* or *Antimonium tartaricum* might be indicated. Extreme forms of vertigo can also fall into this category. There was the typical case of a business-man who had to take a hurried trip to South America; the physical reaction to his fear gave him the sensation that he was standing on top of an open high place and that at any moment he was going to fall off. The journey was so terrifying that he was in agony until it was over. The next time he had to fly he had taken the precaution of visiting the doctor and *Argentum nitricum* turned what would have been a nightmare into a pleasant journey. Much rarer is the patient who has the admittedly illogical but positive sensation that the upper part of his body is made of glass. These infrequent symptoms are best treated with *Thuja*, whereas *Lueticum* is the most frequent cure for the more ordinary complaint of compulsive hand washing.

In taking a case the busy homoeopathic doctor is frequently surprised at how the patient's complaints fit into a single remedy. Not long ago there was a man whose 'gammy' knee was causing him trouble and quite sensibly we gave him *Ruta*. Some time later he came in for more medicine to complete the cure and asked off-handedly, 'By the way these pills couldn't have helped my piles could they? Because, when I first came to see you they were giving me great trouble and are now so much better.' *Ruta* is one of the best pile remedies and it was just the remedy for his painful knee as well. The experienced homoeopathic doctor will not necessarily have to go into every detail to find the right remedy, just as the orthodox physican can spot a case of myxoedema or pernicious anaemia, so the homoeopath will be able to tell in an instant whether it is *Phosphorus* or *Pulsatilla* that the patient requires. Nor is he surprised when on a repeat visit he is told about some other, hitherto unrevealed, symptom which has been improved. These have been described recently as one of the beneficial side effects of homoeopathic therapy.

One does not always have to investigate every symptom mentioned in this chapter for the experienced doctor to prescribe the required drug. The patient's story and mental and physical attitudes themselves will often point in the direction of the needed cure. This is easily confirmed by a few simple questions always so posited so that the doctor does not suggest any ideas. It is essential in a busy clinic that the doctor has as full a knowledge of homoeopathic *materia medica*, and this comes with experience. But even in the early stages doctors acquire a thorough knowledge of quite a small number of remedies which are astonishingly effective.

6

Types of Remedies

However homoeopathic remedies are classified, it is always on the totality of the symptoms that the drug is selected for treatment. The symptoms of acute poisoning by arsenic where diarrhoea and vomiting were so prevalent, were well known in the workshops in Hahnemann's day. The symptoms of chronic poisoning of which Hahnemann was fully aware, were shown in such things as skin rashes, and nervous symptoms. These symptoms came out markedly in the provings upon healthy people even using the potentized remedy. These might be called the outwardly reflected image of the internal and invisible disease.

In acute illness there is little difficulty in determining the totality of the symptoms; for example in flu, the onset is sudden, with a rapid rise of temperature, accompanied by headaches, sore throat, general weakness and aching in the limbs with possibly a cough or stomach upset.

Hahnemann says that whatever one's clinical diagnosis, the therapy must be squarely placed on the ascertainable symptoms and signs. As we have no other guide for prescribing, he emphasizes that we must be particularly and almost exclusively attentive to the symptoms that are peculiar or characteristic of the patient rather than to those that are common to the disease.

As provings increased, it was possible to group remedies into categories, and those that gave a wide range of symptoms in the provers were termed the Polycrests, which include *Sulphur, Pulsatilla, Lycopodium, Phosphorus* etc. These were not classified until Hahnemann was proving medicines in potency. These Polycrests are widely applicable and are particularly useful in chronic illnesses where constitutional prescribing is of most value. A Polycrest in potency is a remedy with a wide range of action affecting all tissues of the body in some degree. Dr Margaret Tyler in her article on *Pulsatilla* (1932) describes it as one of Hahnemann's Polycrests or a drug of many uses. It establishes in its provings symptoms in every part of the body, and she quotes Hahnemann's definition of a Polycrest in provings in her article on *Nux vomica*, so that a Polycrest can be described as a remedy with a wide range of action. It may have an action in one system as is seen in *Sulphur*, which for 2000 years has been used for skin complaints although the homoeopath would look at the whole patient.

There is no doubt that all the Polycrests are constitutional drugs and that the whole make up of the patient must be taken into account and consideration as it always should be in prescribing. The proving of these remedies has also indicated that certain persons produce a fuller picture of the total symptomatology than others, which is due to the individual characteristics of the provers. These are the common things about people which identify them— sociable or unsociable, sensitive to criticism, to music, to noise, to touch—even to a thunder storm. The person who throws an extra log on the fire, and his companion who flings up the window because he must have some air, and when the tea-tray appears pours himself a scalding cup of tea with six lumps of sugar. You will recognize these as general characteristics of a patient which were discussed in the last chapter on taking the case.

The term Polycrest was invented by Hahnemann some time in or about 1817 in his article on *Nux vomica*, in the second volume of his *Materia Medica Pura*, and he wrote 'There are a few medicines the majority of whose symptoms are of the commonest and most frequent occurrence in human diseases, hence very often found in efficacious homoeopathic employment, they are called polycrests'.

A great many substances have been tested, not only familiar substances known to the apothecaries of Hahnemann's day, but an increasing number of others. Those which have been tested have been proved on clinical experience and collected by Dr Clarke.

There are however, several different methods for the classification of drugs. For example, the periodic table is one of the best methods of classifying the elements, which are single substances and not compounds, according to their atomic weight. It is interesting to observe that *Sulphur*, *Tellurium* and *Selenium* follow each other in this classification and show certain parallels in their provings. *Sulphur* is an elementary substance occurring in nature as a brittle crystalline solid, burning with a blue flame when exposed to air. Its reputation as a remedy had been known and used in earliest times as a powerful specific against itch. This power was abused. It was used in baths and local applications, ointments, and, as a result it was found that skin irritations were not cured but rather worsened. Hahnemann found in *Sulphur* the homoeopathic counterpart of the peculiar constitutional bad health (dyscrasia) which tends to show itself in itch-like eruptions and which he named *Psora*.

Tellurium occurs in the natural state in combination with gold, silver, lead and antimony. In its chemical reactions it resembles *Sulphur* and *Selenium*—and was first introduced into homoeopathy by Dr Hering in 1850. In its provings, skin irritations were the most marked symptom and it was used with very good results in *Herpes circinatus*, and had a great reputation in the cure of ringworm, particularly of the face and body. It was also found to be an important remedy in otorrhoea and a principal cure for offensive footsweat when that is included in the whole symptom picture.

The famous pianist Dame Myra Hess, had severe back pain and dreaded the possibility of having her back touched or pressed, she was X-rayed and early arthritis was distinctly shown in her lower back. If her back was pressed in any way, she felt pain going up to her head, and then all over her, so that she could hardly go on. She had to push herself up from the piano-stool after playing. *Tellurium* cured her, and her X-ray plates confirmed this to the amazement of those who had seen her in the early stages.

Selenium was first discovered in 1818—it was found to be associated with *Tellurium* (*tellus* the earth) and *Sulphur* and belonged to the same group of elements. It was introduced and proved by Dr Hering. It is a great remedy for weakness of any kind brought on by hot weather, over-exertion, mental or physical, night-watching etc. The patient regains strength as the sun sinks. His weakness leads to sleepiness, although he feels worse for sleep. Its parallelism with *Sulphur* is shown perfectly on the skin, and can be seen recurring where the ailment and treatment are somewhat similar. The prescription of *Selenium* depends upon the severity of the weakness.

The plants that are used cover an enormous range, and again, were proved on healthy human beings. These did not only include plants that were known like *Belladonna* and

Nux vomica, Ipecacuanha, but many others which are un-familiar such as Sun-Dew (*Drosera*). Club Moss, which was only used at that time as a coating for pills, after being homoeopathically prepared by Hahnemann produced a most powerful drug picture and is in daily use in any homoeopathic practice as *Lycopodium.*

Dr Paterson from Glasgow, who did a lot of work on bowel germs, found that in the ordinary homoeopathic treatment of the patient, the relation between certain groups of organisms changed as the patient improved. He made preparations of bowel flora to restore the balance and very often cured the complaint. Since Paterson's original work, his followers have extended the use of the bowel nosodes beyond that which was established by scientific experiment. The symptomatology of the remedies is found to corres-pond with the symptoms complained of by patients whose bowel flora have become unbalanced.

Many of the patients whom Dr Paterson investigated had already been prescribed for with one of these homoeo-pathic remedies, but there was one who had not responded in the expected way. He then gave the nosode indicated by the examination of the patient's bowel flora which resulted in a very marked improvement. If anything further was needed, it was usually one of the associated remedies. The basic work on these bowel nosodes was done before the antibiotic era and any repetition of this work now is not possible; antibiotics have made such a difference to the bowel flora. But the application of the principles in pre-scribing for chronic ill health is as efficacious as it ever was. Further work on remedies called the bowel nosodes can be very useful. These are prepared from the non-lactose fermenting organisms of the bowel, and are very helpful in two ways. Firstly, they will show by bacteriological exam-ination which of the organisms has become unbalanced, and the nosode itself can often put a patient right. Secondly, it has been found over the last thirty years, largely due to Dr Paterson's work, that certain homoeopathic remedies are closely associated with the different bowel nosodes. Thus, a *Dysentery Co* patient may call for *Lycopodium* or *Arsenicum* or *Nux vomica*, or *Argentum nitricum*.

There is very often a valuable past history of dysentery and the patient may respond perfectly to *Dysentery Co* and need nothing further. A man in out-patients who was brought in a bath-chair completely crippled by rheumatoid arthritis gave a history of never being well since he had dysentery. Though Dr Paterson recommended the 6th potency in such a case, I gave him *Dysentery Co* 30 and in a month came in on two sticks, some weeks later on one stick, and finally he walked without any difficulty. He attended out-patients' for a year once a month and never needed any other remedy, and was back in his old job and doing very well.

A very interesting case was of a patient who had also never been well since a febrile illness and finally, after twenty years of backache and bone pain the diagnosticians found he had in fact got it from typhoid fever. This shows again how an acute illness can leave very puzzling after effects—a fact which the homoeopaths have recognized for years and, moreover, have been able to treat.

The organism *Proteus* is associated with *Secale* and several other remedies. A patient who had an operation for bowel cancer was admitted to hospital as she was so very unwell. On bacterial examination of her stool she was found to have a great excess of *bacillus proteus* and was given *Proteus 30*. She improved at once, and the bacteriologist was extremely interested in the way that the bowel adjusted, and with the fact that she was much better than he had expected.

Bacillus gaertner is associated with the remedies *Phosphorus*, *Silica* and *Mercury*. The patients who come into this group are bright and intelligent but have rather poor bodies—

there may be a history of old coeliac disease found in the colon.

Morgan Co (*Bach*) is another of the bowel nosodes and is associated with *Petroleum*, *Sulphur* and *Psorinum* and is found very useful in chronic gastritis, general congestion in the pelvic organs or defects of circulation—oedema and congestion of the feet and many of the skin complaints. The symptoms must fit the whole picture of the patient but when he is not responding well to other remedies, it is very satisfactory if a nosode applies.

Morgan Co has two sub-types:

1. *Morgan pure*, which seems to be closely associated with *Sulphur* and *Psorinum* and can lift a patient over the next fence when these remedies have not done all that was expected of them.
2. *Morgan gaertner* which bears a close resemblance to *Lycopodium* in the patient's symptoms, and which can give great relief in a patient who is not doing as well as one would expect on his definite constitutional remedy *Lycopodium*.

At the time of the discovery of the tuberculosis germ, which had been met with great interest, a successful vaccine against rabies had also been found. The same principle, used successfully against hydrophobia, was applied to tuberculosis bacillus, but unfortunately a number of patients died because of the toxicity. Dr Compton-Burnett's preparation of the culture of the organisms made according to homoeopathic principles removed all danger of the toxicity and was found to cure many tubercular patients.

The principle of vaccine therapy had already been established homoeopathically. Even the treatment of rabies had been made possible in the United States not only by Dr Hering but by Dr Swann who had prepared a potency from the saliva of a rabid dog which he called *Lyssin*. This valuable use of the actual disease products, called isopathy, has not been sufficiently recognized in recent historical surveys of the history of bacteriology.

The influenza viruses have proved extremely useful in potentized form as a prophylactic against epidemic influenza and fevers, borne out by the use of homoeopathic anti-cold and flu pills. These are particularly useful as preventive medicines if taken regularly between September and March. It is singularly useful for people such as heads of state, politicians, lecturers and actors who are committed well in advance to a heavy schedule of public engagements. It has not been possible to prove in the laboratory that the antibodies are raised, but in a clinical situation, thousands of people have found that these remedies indeed cure, or prevent, frequent colds and influenza. Although these nosodes have proved helpful in preventing recurrent infection, in treatment the homoeopathic remedy must be founded again on the totality of the symptoms.

As the science of bacteriology developed further, and viruses were isolated, their pure organisms were made into potencies and used as prophylactics and therapeutic agents. These have not been proved in a truly homoeopathic sense but are an addition to the homoeopathic pharmacopoeia, and there is no limit to the number of microorganisms which can be included. We have now achieved clinical results over the last forty years so that these agents are being used in a clinical situation which present similar symptoms to the disease with which the organism is associated.

The early homoeopaths also investigated the poisonous effects of spider and insect bites and stings and extracted these to make up a potency. Snake venoms have been extracted and used for many years and Dr Hering's preparation of *Lachesis* (from the bushmaster) was one of the first to be discovered.

The *Tarentula* (the poison from any one of the different tarantula spider family) picture is one of mental excitement and hysteria accompanied by all sorts of hallucinations together with rage and fury. A girl with an appendix abscess wanted to be left alone in the dark; if disturbed she would burst into a fury, and said how easy it would be to fall out of the sixth floor window to end it all. Because of these changes of mood and her strange desires she was given *Tarentula*. There was no further trouble and she was quite calm through an operation and subsequent treatment.

The value of trace elements upon the body's physiology is only now being investigated. Among the first discoveries to be investigated was the importance of cobalt with zinc. But zinc, magnesium and copper are trace elements found to be invaluable in small quantities in the cellular responses. For some time, it has been recognized that *Calcium* and *Chloride* were involved in fluid balance—it has been known for a long time that anaemia is associated with iron deficiency. All these trace elements are in the homoeo-pathic *Materia Medica* and have been found to produce a symptom picture which in many respects may resemble the type of problems associated with the deficiency.

At one time nobody could link the clinical picture of the symptoms of sway-back in sheep, where the animal could not walk straight or balance, and up to very recently these animals had to be destroyed. But modern scientific experimentation, following precisely those lines laid down by Hahnemann in the eighteenth century—with no clinical thermometer, sphygmomanometer, microscope or stetho-scope—of observation and notation, has now revealed that the disease is caused by a deficiency of copper. Copper, is, as we know, one of the metals which falls into a homoeopathic classification.

Apart from the provings of drugs on healthy individuals, we come to the susceptibility and toxicological effects on animals. Although as yet this field has not been subject to the research as extensively as it should be, we do have some examples of animals proving symptoms.

As an example, sheep which graze beneath Mount Hecla are very apt to get bony swellings on their backs and around their joints—when this condition is met with in patients it can be treated with potentized *Hecla lava* with good results.

Through the years I have seen bony spurs on the feet removed by this, and a family with diaphysial aclasia responded well. It is often useful in Paget's disease which is an enlargement of the bone.

In animals eating Bryonia plants, a pleural effusion can occur in the chest, and this can be one of the common remedies for pleurisy.

In his book *Principles and Practice*, Dr Wheeler wrote, 'Chronic disease is chronic mainly because of a failure on the part of the system involved to carry resistance through to victory. If the structures involved are not immediately essential to life, or if there is enough relatively normal remaining then the curious economy of our bodies appears to tolerate the presence of disease.'

In the prescription of drugs it is important to note that as soon as definite improvement of the symptoms sets in, the administration of the remedy should be stopped, and as long as improvement continues no further doses should be given.

Just as there are many different characteristics in a general illness so there are many possible remedies. Take as a classification *The Cold Remedies*. These include *Arsenicum album*, *Nitric acid*, *Hepar sulphuris* and *Nux vomica*. These are all remedies for patients who feel the cold intensely. All four remedies have hyperaesthesia although it affects them in different ways.

Arsenicum album is oversensitive to her surroundings, to smell, touch, having hair combed—and with it some degree of anxiety, and an anxious expression.

Nitric acid is particularly sensitive to physical disturbances —he is upset beyond reason by hip pain or pain elsewhere, and is very sensitive to touch.

Hepar sulphuris has marked cutaneous hyperaesthesia, especially to touch, draught, but also to personal atmosphere. He is easily upset, and apt to fly into a temper.

Nux vomica has more cutaneous sensitiveness than the rest—not so much to pain but to cold, touch, noise, being disturbed or interfered with in any way, and appears very startled if touched suddenly, his nerves on edge.

All four are worse when alone:

Arsenicum album afraid of anything and apt to panic in the night, often likes a night-light, is worse alone, and worse between mid-night and 1 am, will worry not only about self, but everything else around.

Nitric acid always has a certain amount of fear alone, often a deep fear of death.

Hepar sulphuris nothing like the *Arsenicum* patient's fear of being alone, but has a reaction of great irritability to being alone for long and is definitely nervous.

Nux vomica definite business anxiety when alone, about money, or whether he'll be fit to do his job; not the acute fear of *Arsenicum* patient, but very often accompanied by some underlying anxiety about his health.

All four are impulsive to an unusual extent:

Arsenicum album worse in times of stress—impulsiveness works up to an acute state of apprehension, sometimes cannot stand it any longer and may even feel like attempting suicide.

Nitric acid not so impulsive as others of the group.

Hepar sulphuris impulsive and quarrelsome—exhibition of temper at sight of certain people, if annoyed sufficiently, particularly in children; they will kick and hit, and possibly do real damage.

Nux vomica like *Arsenicum* and *Hepar* but to a much lesser degree.

All four tend to have a liking for fat:

Arsenicum album generally has a liking for fat, but once in a while loses his craving for it.

Nitric acid likes and desires fat, although he may get an aggravation from taking it and digestive symptoms.

Hepar sulphuris likes fat, but knows that it will upset him and usually avoids it in consequence.

Nux vomica likes fat very much, and digests it well.

All four have some swallowing difficulty:

Arsenicum album complains that food sticks and causes choking, coughing and spluttering; food may come up.

Nitric acid gets choking, sticking pain as if food refuses to go down.

Hepar sulphuris feeling of something stuck in the throat which may be very painful.

Nux vomica feels that food goes down the oesophagus quite a long way, then becomes very uncomfortable and food returns, not connected with pain, more as if peristaltic action had gone the wrong way.

All tend to be somewhat better in rainy weather:

Arsenicum album tends to be very, very chilly and is often worse on a cold dry day, and may be better in gentle rain.

Nitric acid is worse in cold dry weather and often says he is better in damp.

Hepar sulphuris is very sensitive to cold, particularly to cold windy weather and is often better in rain.

Nux vomica is worse in dry cold weather but definitely better on rainy days.

There are several classifications of remedies and I would like to mention here, one of the best known, that done by Dr Boyd of Glasgow. He classified drugs according to their electro-physical properties. He discovered that a patient tends to remain constantly in his own group throughout life so long as the normal balance of health is maintained. When the health becomes unbalanced from conditions which are not acute, the tendency is to change into a group of a related series. So that, for an example, someone normally defined as a member of group 1 might change and belong to group 6 or 10. The most common series consists of groups 1, 6 and 10.

Unfortunately Dr. Boyd died before completing his work, nevertheless his groupings are of importance.

GROUP 1

Acon. (*Aconitum napellus*); monk's hood
Brom. (*Bromium*); bromine
Calc. brom. (*Calcarea bromata*)
Chlor. (*Chlorinum*)
Cobalt. (*Cobaltum metallicum*)
Cyclamen
Ferr. Brom. (*Ferrum bromatum*)
Ferr. Met. (*Ferrum metallicum*)
Ferr. Mur. (*Ferrum muriaticum*)
Glon. (*Glonoin*); nitroglycerine

Guaiac (*Guaiacum officinale*); lignum vitae
Manchineel (*Mancinella hippomane*)
Oleander (*Nerium oleander*)
Oleum an. (*Oleum animale aethereum*); Dippel's animal oil
Oleum jec. (*Oleum jecoris aselli*); cod liver oil
Sepia (*Sepia officinalis*) cuttlefish ink
Verat. alb. (*Veratrum album*); European hellebore
Verat. vir. (*Veratrum viride*); American hellebore

GROUP 2

Aur. brom. (*Aurum bromatum*)
Aur. met. (*Aurum metallicum*); gold
Aur. mur. (*Aurum muriaticum*)
Aur. sulph. (*Aurum sulphuratum*)
Bothrops (*Bothrops lanceolatus*)
Calc. met. (*Calcarea metallica*)
Cenchris (*Cenchris contortrix*)
Crotal. hor. (*Crotalus horridus*); rattle-snake venom
Elaps (*Elaps corallinus*); coral snake
Heloderma (*Heloderma horridus*); gila monster

Hura (*Hura brasiliensis*), sand box tree
Lach. (*Lachesis muta*); bushmaster
Murex (*Murex purpurea*); sea gastropod
Naja (*Naja tripudians*); cobra
Squid
Sting Ray
Sysig. (*Syzygium jambolanum*)
Toxicoph; poison, Mocassin snake venom
Trombid. (*Trombidium muscae domesticae*); house fly; mites
Vipera (*Vipera torva*); viper

GROUP 3

Alfalfa

T.N.T.

GROUP 4

Aesculus (*Aesculus hippocastanum*);
   horse chestnut
Ammon. carb. (*Ammonium car-*
   bonicum)
Ammon.   mur.   (*Ammonium*
   muriaticum)
Badiaga; fresh water sponge
Bar. carb. (*Baryta carbonica*); barium
   carbonate
Bar. met. (*Baryta metallicum*)
Bry. (*Bryonia alba*)
Caladium (*Caladium seguinum*)
Calc. Acet. (*Calcarea acetica*)
Calc. carb. (*Calcarea carbonica*)
Calc. chlor. (*Calcarea chloratum*)
Calc. fluor. (*Calcarea fluorica*)
Calc.   hypo.   phos.   (*Calcarea*
   hypophosphorica)
Calc. lact (*Calcarea lactica*)
Calc. ovi testis (*Calcarea ovi testae*)
Calc. oxal. (*Calcarea oxalica*)
Card. mar. (*Carduus marianus*); thistle
Con. (*Conium*); poison hemlock
Coryza

Digit. (*Digitalis purpurea*); foxglove
Dulc. (*Dulcamara*); woody night-
   shade
Equis. (*Equisetum hyemale*); horsetail
Fluor.   ac.   (*Acidum   fluoricum*);
   hydrofluoric acid
Ign. (*Ignatia amara*); similar to
   strychnine
Millefol.   (*Achillea   millefolium*);
   yarrow
Mosch.   (*Moschus   tunquinensis*);
   musk
Myosotis (*Myosotis symphitifolia*);
   forget-me-not
Onos. (*Onosmodium virginianum*)
Opojex
Ovar. res. T.
Parathyroid M.
Podo.   (*Podophyllum   peltatum*);
   American mandrake
Sars. (*Sarsaparilla*)
Sinap. (*Sinapis nigra*); mustard
Thyroid
Viburnum (*Viburnum opulus*)

GROUP 5

Acet. acid (*Acidum aceticum*)
Act. spicata (*Actea spicata*); bane-
   berry
Adrenalin
Agnus. cast. (*Agnus castus*);
Aloe (*Aloe socotrina*)
Alumina
Alum. met. (*Aluminium metallicum*)
Alum. phos. (*Aluminium phosphori-*
   cum)
Apis (*Apis mellifica*); honey-bee
Arg. met. (*Argentum metallicum*); silver
Arg. nit. (*Argentum nitricum*)
Arum trip. (*Arum triphyllum*)
Bell. (*Belladonna*)
Benz. ac. (*Acidum benzoicum*)
Bovista   (*Lycoperdon   giganteum*);
   giant puffball

Cad. lact. (*Cadmium lacticum*)
Cad.   nat.   sil.   fluor.   (*Cadmium*
   natrum silicea fluoricum)
Cad. phos. (*Cadmium phosphoricum*)
Cad. sil. (*Cadmium silicate*)
Cajaput.   (*Cajaputi*);   California
   laurel
Calc. phos. (*Calcarea phosphorica*)
Cann. ind. (*Cannabis indica*)
Cann. sat. (*Cannabis sativa*)
Carb. acid (*Acidum carbolicum*)
Carcin. (*Carcinosinum*); cancer nosode
Ceanoth
China. (*China officinalis*)
Chloral. (*Chloralum*)
Clematis (*Clematis erecta*)
Cimic.   (*Cimicifuga   racemosa*);
   bugbane, snake root

Chrom. met. (*Chromium metallicum*)
Cina
Coccus cacti
Condurango; condor vine
Cupressus (*Cupressus lawsonia*)
    cypress
Cuprum(*Cuprum metallicum*); copper
Elat. (*Elaterium*), squirting
    cucumber
Fago. (*Fagopyrum esculentum*);
    buckwheat
Ferr. phos. (*Ferrum phosphoricum*)
Fragaria (*Fragaria vesca*); straw-
    berry
Genoscop
Iris t. (*Iris tenax*)
Iris v. (*Iris versicolor*)
Influenzin (*Influenzinum*)
Juglans (*Juglans regia*); walnut
Kalmia (*Kalmia latifolia*); laurel
Lac. acid. (*Acidum lacticum*); soured
    milk
Lac. can. (*Lac caninum*)
Lact. sat. (*Lactuca sativa*); garden
    lettuce
Lact. vir. (*Lactuca virosa*)
Ledum (*Ledum palustre*); Labrador
    Tea
Lept. (*Leptandra virginica*); Culver's
    physic
Lil. tig. (*Lilium tigrinum*)
Lobelia (*Lobelia inflata*)
Lycop. (*Lycopodium clavatum*); club
    moss
Mag. mur. (*Magnesia muriatica*)
Mag. phos. (*Magnesia phosphorica*)
Manganum (*Manganum metallicum*)
Melilotus (*Melilotus officinalis*);
    sweet clover
Mur. acid. (*Acidum muriaticum*)
Myrica (*Myrica cerifera*); bayberry
Myrtus. com. (*Myrtus communis*);
    myrtle
Nat. benz. (*Natrum benzoicum*)
Nat. bicarb. (*Natrum bicarbonicum*)

Nat. brom. (*Natrum bromicum*)
Nat. carb. (*Natrum carbonicum*)
Nat. lac. (*Natrum lacticum*)
Nat. mur. (*Natrum muriaticum*)
Nat. oleate. (*Natrum oleate*)
Nat. phos. (*Natrum phosphoricum*)
Nat. salicyl. (*Natrum salicylicum*)
Nat. sil. (*Natrum silicum*)
Neosalvarsan (Bayer)
Nux mosch. (*Nux moschata*)
Orchic (*Orchitinum*)
Ornithogalum (*Ornithogalum
    umbellatum*); star of bethlehem
Oxal. acid. (*Acidum oxalicum*); salt
    of lemons
Pallad. (*Palladium metallicum*)
Phos. (*Phosphorus*)
Phos. ac. (*Acidum phosphoricum*)
Phyt. (*Phytolacca decandra*); poke
    weed
Plumb. (*Plumbum metallicum*)
Ran. bulb. (*Ranunculus bulbosus*)
Ran. scler. (*Ranunculus sceleratus*)
Raphanus (*Raphanus sativus*);
    radish
Sabad. (*Sabadilla*)
Scarlatinum (*Scarlatinum*)
Scirrin (*Scirrhinum*)
Secale. (*Secale cornutum*); ergot
    mould
Senecio (*Senecio aureus*); groundsel
Solan. Tub. a. (*Solanum tuberosum
    aegrotans*); potato (diseased)
Spig. (*Spigelia anthelmintica*)
Staph. (*Staphisagria*); larkspur
Stront. carb. (*Strontiana carbonica*)
Sulph. acid. (*Acidum sulphuricum*)
S.U.P.
Suprarenal cortex
Tabac. (*Tabacum*)
Therid. (*Theridion curassavicum*);
    spider
Uric acid (*Acidum uricum*)
Ustilago (*Ustilago maidis*); corn-
    smut

Vespa (*Vespa crabro*); the wasp

Wyethia (*Wyethia helenoides*)

GROUP 6

Allium cepa; onion
Anac. (*Anacardium orientale*); marking nut
Anthracinum
Ant. Ars. (*Antimonium arsenicum*)
Ant. crudum (*Antimonium crudum*)
Ant. tart. (*Antimonium tartaricum*)
Aranea (*Aranea diadema*); spider
Ars. alb. (*Arsenicum album*)
Ars. met. (*Arsenicum metallicum*)
Arundo (*Arundo mauritanica*); reeds
Bapt. (*Baptisia tinctoria*); indigo
Bismuthum (*Bismuthum metallicum*)
Cact. grand. (*Cactus grandiflora*)
Cad. ars. (*Cadmium arsenicum*)
Cad. met. (*Cadmium metallicum*)
Cad. mur. (*Cadmium muriaticum*)
Cad. sulph. (*Cadmium sulphuratum*)
Calc. ars. (*Calcarea arsenicosa*)
Calc. caust. (*Calcarea caustica*)
Calc. sil. (*Calcarea silicata*)
Capsicum (*Capsicum annuum*); green pepper
Caust. (*Causticum*)
Cedron (*Cedron simaba*); rattlesnake bean
Cocculus (*Cocculus indicus*); moonseed
Coral. rub. (*Corallium rubrum*); red coral
Crataegus oxy. (*Crataegus oxyacantha*); hawthorn
Crocus (*Crocus sativus*)
Curare
Echi. (*Echinacea angustifolia*); rudbeckia

Euphrasia (*Euphrasia officinalis*); eyebright
Ferr. ars. (*Ferrum arseniatum*)
Gels. (*Gelsemium sempervirens*); jasmine
Graph. (*Graphites*)
Gratiola (*Gratiola officinalis*); hyssop
Hydrocyan. ac. (*Acidum hydrocyanicum*)
Hyper. (*Hypericum perforatum*); St. John's wort
Kali mur. (*Kali muriaticum*)
Kali nit. (*Kali nitricum*)
Lapis alb. (*Lapis albus*)
Lith. carb. (*Lithium carbonicum*)
Malaria
Mephitis; skunk
Nat. ars. (*Natrum arsenicosum*)
Pareira (*Pareira brava*); moonseed drug
Pituit. post (T)
Pitglandis (T)
Samb. (*Sambucus nigra*); elder
Sang. (*Sanguinaria canadiensis*); bloodroot
Spong. (*Spongia tosta*); sponge
Squil. (*Squilla maritima*)
Sticta. (*Sticta pulmonaria*); lichen
Tarent. (*Tarentula cubensis*); spider poison, Cuban tarantula
Teuc. mar. ver. (*Teucrium marum verum*)
Verbasc. (*Verbascum thapsus*); figwort
Vinca (*Vinca minor*); periwinkle
Viola (*Viola odorata*)

GROUP 7

Arsen. iod. (*Arsenicum iodatum*)
Kali ars. (*Kalium arsenicosum*)
Kali car. (*Kalium carbonicum*)
Lac. deflor. (*Lac defloratum*); skimmed milk

Lachnan. (*Lachnanthes tinctoria*); Red root
Nuphar lut. (*Nuphar luteum*); water lily
Syph. (*Syphilinum*)
Thea (*Thea chinensis*); tea

GROUP 8

Agar. (*Agaricus muscarius*); fly agaric

Aphis. chen. glauc. (*Aphis chenopodii glauci*); aphid

Aralia. (*Aralia racemosa*); angelica

Artemisia (*Artemisia vulgaris*)

Bach's Intestinal Nosodes

Bacillinum

Berb. (*Berberis vulgaris*)

Bufo. (*Bufo cinereus*); toad

Cad. calc. iod. (*Cadmium calcarea iodata*)

Cad. iod. (*Cadmium iodata*)

Calc. iod. (*Calcarea iodata*)

Canth. (*Cantharis vesicatoria*); beetle, spanish-fly

Carbo. an. (*Carbo animalis*)

Carbo. veg. (*Carbo vegetabilis*)

Carbo. sulph. (*Carbo sulphuratum*)

Cauloph. (*Caulophyllum thalictroides*); barberry

Cham. (*Chamomilla*)

Chel. (*Chelidonium majus*); celandine

Chenopod. anth. (*Chenopodium anthelminticum*); pigweed

Chimaphil. (*Chimaphila umbellata*); prince's pine

China acid. (*Chininum acidicum*)

China sulph. (*Chininum sulphuricum*)

Cicuta (*Cicuta virosa*); poison parsley

Coffea (*Coffea cruda*); wild coffee

Colch. (*Colchicum autumnale*); autumn crocus

Coloc. (*Colocynthis*); bitter apple

Diosc. (*Dioscorea villosa*); the yam

Dirca (*Dirca palustris*); swamp-wood

Dros. (*Drosera*); sundew

Egg white

Eup. per. (*Eupatorium perfoliatum*); boneset

Ferr. iod. (*Ferrum iodatum*)

Gnaphal. (*Gnaphalium polycephalum*); cudweed

Gunpowder

Hamamelis (*Hamamelis virginiana*); American witch hazel

Hydrastis (*Hydrastis canadensis*); golden seal, Indiana turmeric

Indigo

Iod. (*Iodum*)

Ipec. (*Ipecacuanha*)

Kali bich. (*Kalium bichromicum*)

Kali brom. (*Kalium bromatum*)

Kali chlor. (*Kalium chloricum*)

Kali iod. (*Kalium iodatum*)

Kali met. (*Kalium metallicum*)

Kali sulph. (*Kalium sulphuricum*)

Koch's cancer serum

Kreosote

Latrodectus mact. (*Latrodectus modans*), black widow spider

Lyssin

Mag. carb. (*Magnesia carbonica*)

Mag. sulph. (*Magnesia sulphurica*)

Malandrinum; sallenders

Medorrhinum

Menyanthis (*Menyanthes trifoliata*); the buck-bean

Merc. cyan. (*Mercurius cyanatus*)

Merc. dulc. (*Mercurius dulcis*)

Merc. iod. flav. (*Mercurius iodatus flavus*)

Merc. iod. rub. (*Mercurius iodatus ruber*)

Merc. sol. (*Mercurius solubilis*)

Merc. sulph. (*Mercurius sulphuricus*)

Merc. viv. (*Mercurius vivus*)

Mez. (*Mezereum*)

Morph. acet. (*Morphinum acetatum*)

Nat. iod. (*Natrum iodatum*)

Nat. sul. (*Natrum sulphuricum*)

Nux. vom. (*Nux vomica*); strychnine

Oenanthe (*Oenanthe crocata*); water dropwort

Opium

Oxytropis (*Oxytropis lamberti*); loco-weed

Petrol. (*Petroleum*)

Petros. (*Petroselinum sativum*); parsley

Phelland. (*Phellandrium aquaticum*)

Picric. acid. (*Acidum picricum*)

Platinum (*Platinum metallicum*)

Prunus (*Prunus spinosa*); sloe

Psor. (*Psorinum*); itch

Puls. (*Pulsatilla vulgaris*); pasque-flower

Pyrogen (*Pyrogenium*)

Rad. brom. (*Radium bromatum*)

Rhod. (*Rhododendron chrysanthum*);

Rhus. tox. (*Rhus toxicodendron*); poison ivy

Ruta (*Ruta graveolens*); rue

Scleros (*Sclerosin*)

Selenium (*Selenium metallicum*)

Senega; snake root

S.S.C. (*Sulphur, Silicea, Carbo vegetabilis*)

GROUP 9

Borax (*Natrum biborate*)

Gallium (*Gallium metallicum*)

GROUP 10

Arnica (*Arnica montana*)

Calc. sulph. (*Calcarea sulphurica*)

China ars. (*Chininum arsenicosum*)

Cistus (*Cistus canadensis*); rock-rose

Helleborus N. (*Helleborus niger*); Christmas rose

Helleborus V. (*Helleborus viridis*); Lenten rose

Hepar. Sulph. (*Hepar sulphuris calcarea*)

GROUP 11

Asafoetida

Asarum (*Asarum europaeum*); asara-bacca

Calotropis (*Calotropis gigantea*); milkweed

Helonias (*Helonias dioica*)

GROUP 12

Valeriana (*Valeriana officinalis*)

Stannum (*Stannum metallicum*); tin

Stramonium (*Datura stramonium*); thorn apple

Sulphur

Sulph. iod. (*Sulphur iodatum*)

Sumbul (*Sumbulus moschatus*); musk root

Sycotic Co (Paterson)

Symphoricarpus (*Symphoricarpus racemosus*); snowberry

Taraxacum (*Taraxacum officinale*); dandelion

Tellurium (*Tellurium metallicum*)

Tereb. (*Terebenum*); turpentine

Variolinum; smallpox

Viscum alb. (*Viscum album*); European mistletoe

Zinc

Zinc mur. (*Zincum muriaticum*).

Zinc sulph. (*Zincum sulphuricum*)

Gambogia (*Gummi gutti*); gamboge

Sabina (*Juniperus sabina*); juniper

Hippoz. (*Hippozaenin*)

Laurocerasus (*Prunus laurocerasus*); Cherry laurel

Nitric acid (*Acidum nitricum*)

Osmium

Plantago (*Plantago major*); plantain

Rheum (*Rheum palmatum*); rhubarb

Symphitum (*Symphytum officinale*); comfrey

Tuberculinum

Uranium nit. (*Uranium nitricum*)

Paeonia (*Paeonia officinalis*); paeony

Solan. nig. (*Solanum nigrum*)

Stillingia (*Stillingia sylvatica*); queen's delight .

Thallium (*Thallium metallicum*)

Thall. acet. (*Thallium acetate*)

Thuja(*Thuja occidentalis*); arbor vitae

7

The Homoeopathic Materia Medica

Hahnemann called his *Materia Medica* by the term 'pure' indicating that it was not merely conjectural but that the drugs had been proved. His followers continued to maintain his ideals. If a homoeopath wants to investigate a particular drug he must start by getting it proved, and proved by as many people as possible. These people must be thoroughly healthy, old enough to report accurately on the symptoms which occur and not too old to have been damaged in any way by drugs or faulty diet.

Many remedies have been thoroughly proved and have shown their usefulness in clinical experience. Others have not had full proving but are known to be useful in certain conditions. It is perfectly evident that the deliberate taking of remedies by healthy individuals must stand as the most important source of our *materia medica*. At the same time a good deal of knowledge has been accumulated from the effect of drugs taken accidentally or otherwise. Examination will reveal the pathological changes which can be produced by an agent used as a homoeopathic medicine. It is nevertheless more valuable to follow the symptoms produced in the proving of the effect of small doses given to individuals over some time than to prescribe on the effect of massive doses. It is on this base of prolonged experience over many years in comparing many cases, that the homoeopath can have confidence that the treatment given for early symptoms does ward off the more pronounced symptoms that would otherwise follow. It is for this reason that the symptoms produced by provings are preferable to those produced by poisoning.

It has been said that symptoms recorded by provers might have arisen from the effect of all the attention and expectation that they met with when trying to make these reports, and that they are not drug effects at all. This was foreseen by Hahnemann and the early provers, and they tried to eliminate this possibility by not identifying the substance being proved and by their strenuous cross-examination of each prover. They threw out doubtful symptoms and found that a symptom would be repeated by several provers and so verified. They also recognized that some provers were more sensitive to a drug than others and could give genuine and most valuable symptoms which others could miss. The final proof of the test comes in choosing the remedy for the actual case. If any symptom given proves a help in the choice of a remedy (as shown by a disappearance of a marked symptom after giving the drug) then that counts as a confirmation for the truth of that symptom in the proving.

In establishing a proving of a possible remedy, we are considering the symptoms of an ailment and the cure. If during the course it is discovered that in many instances, but not necessarily all, a particular symptom disappears then we must consider the remedy as a possible choice when analysing the constitutional whole of a particular patient.

When Hahnemann began to investigate the truth of his discovery he used remedies in material doses not in potencies, and certainly not the massive does given by most of his contemporaries with which he anyhow disagreed. But, he also used only a single drug at any one time in no very great quantity. In searching for a remedy he first sought those whose symptoms of proving and disease were similar, for instance in treating acute diarrhoea he might advocate *Arsenicum alb.* itself as the most indicated treatment. However he soon found that his patients, although ultimately relieved, got an aggravation of their symptoms which he considered undesirable. He therefore began to give smaller and smaller doses and found that most drugs given 'homoeopathically' in quantities that would have been considered negligible seemed very effective. Tinctures were prepared from medicinal plants and the homoeopaths asked for the whole of the plant to be used from root to flower, preferably in the flowering season, by the pharmacists who were expert at preparing the tinctures. The strongest possible tincture made in this way is called the Mother Tincture and is symbolized by the Greek letter φ—successive dilutions or potencies were made from this on the centesimal scale or the decimal. (Potencies are prescribed by No. 1, 3, 6, 12, 30, 200 etc.) No. 1 consists of 1 drop of tincture to 99 drops of the neutral fluid, usually spirits of wine with a small quantity of water. A drop of No. 1 with a further 99 drops of the medium is the second potency—a drop of this and 99 drops of the medium is the third and so on as far as the physician desires. Each successive potency should receive the most thorough succussion and agitation so as to distribute the tincture evenly through the whole of the diluting medium. In the second (decimal) series the steps were made by tens instead of hundreds. Thus the first decimal potency, a 1x, consists of 1 drop of tincture with 9 drops of spirits of wine and water shaken up together. Then one drop of this with 9 drops of alcohol and water gives the second decimal or 2x and so on.

Speaking generally potencies from the tincture to the third centesimal (or 6x) are classified as low potencies, from 3–12 as medium and from 12 or 15 upwards as high, ranging to very high potencies such as 200, 1m and 10m. The problem to the materialistic scientist is that it is impossible to measure the presence of these molecules in the potency and yet we know that the remedy has an effect on the living organism which is often more striking in higher than in lower potencies although of similar nature.*

The very basis of homoeopathy consists of a knowledge of the effect of drugs on healthy people and the practical application of all this work is the ability to select, out of all the remedies known the one and only *simillimum*, that is the remedy whose *materia medica* most closely compares with the symptom-complex of the patient being treated. This is not always easy and requires both study and patience, but for a century and a half there has been a record of the practical experience of many homoeopathic doctors, and from this a beginner can learn and benefit if he so desires.

Many of the remedies of our pharmacopoeia have had exhaustive tests done, but it is probable, and to be hoped, that further investigation will be carried out to add something more of value to many of the provings. There are also many gaps due to certain substances and plants not having yet been fully proved, but which have been found effective after prolonged clinical experience. The homoeopathic physician knows the symptom complex of a good many of these drugs so well that he can choose a remedy with confidence and find it effective.

* See Appendix 1 for a more detailed explanation.

We all know the importance of physical signs in making a diagnosis, but these are not of the first importance in choosing a remedy. It is the individual responses to outside influences (wet, dry, cold or heat, noise etc.) that are the things that guide in one's choice.

In cases of acute disease—pneumonia, acute rheumatism, gastric ulcer—there are wide choices of remedies. But when tissue involvement is present it is seldom that the choice of remedy is a wide one. Some physicians would recommend tinctures or low potencies here and a remedy like *Ornithogalum* tincture given in 5 drops doses after meals in gastric ulcer can clear up the case completely. On the other hand remedies like *Graphites* or *Anacardium* and others may be needed and will do best in high potencies.

In acute diseases there are often only a few symptoms apart from the actual physical signs of disease. Where there is definite tissue involvement, a prescription which fits the whole patient must be found to repair the condition and the damage. Even here there will be room for some choice. *Phosphorus*, *Bryonia* and *Hepar sulph*. all have claims to repair tissue damage in pneumonia and the choice will rest on the presence or absence of some less obvious symptoms. In gastric ulcer the choice may be between *Arsenicum album*, *Graphites* or *Ornithogalum*. In acute rheumatism again *Bryonia* may be needed or such remedies as *Rhus toxicodendron* and *Pulsatilla*. There may be a further choice in some cases where more wide-spread symptoms are obtained.

The potency in which these drugs are given depends on the choice and experience of the physician. Here the homoeopathic physicians vary a lot, some use mainly low potencies and others mainly high. I always think that it depends somehow on the doctor who is looking for a certain rate of improvement in the patient. Also it depends on how responsive the patient is to the disease process such as in a smouldering type of illness like sub-acute rheumatism or in rapid food poisoning with its acute vomiting. Here one must match one's potency to the vital force of the patient as one observes his response to one's treatment and gains in experience. It is essential to know the natural course of a disease in assessing the response to treatment and which potency is likely to be of the greatest value.

It has already been mentioned that homoeopathic physicians vary a good deal in the choice of potency in prescribing for patients. Some use high potencies almost exclusively and others prefer low potencies for their general use. Most of them admit that in acute illness results are quicker with high potencies and are indeed often spectacular. In these cases it is advisable to repeat the remedy constantly in the acute stage and when improvement has really set in cut down the frequency of the dose and stop it altogether when improvement seems certain and is progressive. In chronic cases there is again a difference in the method of administering the homoeopathic drug. There are physicians who feel more confident in using high potencies. In these cases some will use a single dose only and leave it working for as long as improvement continues. Others use 3 or 4 doses all to be taken within 24 hours. These really act in the same way as a single dose but prevent the occasional aggravation which at times can be severe, that can follow one dose. In either method there should be no repeat of a high potency until it is obvious that it has done all it will.

There are times when all physicians use low potencies as tinctures of substances like *Crataegus* and *Ornithogalum* or as low potencies for local symptoms. In such cases as rheumatoid arthritis there are certain drugs known to be particularly effective for specific joints. *Sanguinaria* for a shoulder joint; *Ruta* or *Pulsatilla* particularly for the knee; *Rhus toxicodendron* for lumbago, jaw or any place where there is relief from continuous movement; *Calcarea hypophos.* for hands and wrists; *Natrum phosph.* for elbows; the cadmium salts for the upper back and many others. In such complaints as constipation *Bryonia* or *Nux vomica* or *Opium* or *Alumina* can be very effective taken after meals. *Arnica* is a great standby for fatigue particularly after travelling and stress and it can also be given in low potency for after effects of accidents or bruising where the high potency has been given at the time of the injury but there is still stiffness and discomfort to be cleared up.

There is still need for extensive experiment and observation. It has been suggested that for every case there is an optimum dosage just as there is an optimum remedy but the factors that should help to decide our choice will be firstly the constitution of the patient, because some individuals are so much more sensitive than others, and then one must consider the nature of the drug and whether it produces a sensitive proving or not. Another factor is the nature of the illness, whether it is mainly a gross tissue affection such as an ulcer or an interference with the metabolic processes of the body.

There is no way yet of giving full value to any of these factors, and continued cautious experiment must go on.

There are certain rules here to be taken into account: If a remedy is well indicated by a close resemblance between the picture of the drug proving and the disease it is recommended to give a high potency and to watch the effect of each dose. If a remedy is well indicated but fails, the physician can try other potencies (either higher or lower) before changing the medicine. If the resemblance between drug and disease is not well marked and particularly where it is found that one tissue is seriously affected so that it can be said that the drug has an affinity for that tissue, it is obviously recommended by some physicians that tinctures or low potencies should be chiefly used and repeated regularly. Probably there is a use and a place for all potencies and it is essential for the homoeopathist to be open minded, swift to experiment and patient and careful in recording his results and coming to definite conclusions and he must constantly test out the validity of these conclusions.

There are two further points for consideration—where in acute cases symptoms are few, and chiefly due to tissue involvement. There are definite indications that certain drugs enhance specific processes of body resistance—*Arsenicum* is found to be a general stimulant to phagocytes—*Veratrum viride* raises the opsonic index to the pneumococcus, *Phosphorus* to the tubercle bacillus, *Hepar sulph.* to staphylococcus aureus and *Baptisia* increases the agglutinating power of blood serum towards the typhoid bacillus. In addition homoeopaths used potencies made from disease products even before vaccine therapy had become general and as vaccination procedures developed further the use of potencies of 'nosodes' was also expanded.

Potencies of tubercle, influenza and cold germs pneumococcus and many others were used frequently to obtain similar effects to those arrived at by the injections of laboratory vaccines. There is ample evidence to show the good results obtained, and so nosodes can be given when a bacteriological diagnosis has been made or the drug should be given which is known to affect the specific resistance mechanism. Thus a nosode can be given at this stage and watched with care. It has been found that nosodes may be used in acute conditions when most physicians would hesitate to inject the more 'massive' dose of the ordinary vaccine. The use of *Baptisia* in typhoid or *Veratrum viride* in pneumonia must be guided by the characteristic symptom complexes that these drugs show and should not be given on pathological grounds only. Experience shows that if they are needed for recovery they will be indicated by the symptoms shown in their provings—nosodes are given with less exactitude because so many of them are relatively unproved. On the other hand *Tuberculinum* and *Lueticum* and one or two others which have been known and used on long clinical experience have worked out a kind of proving and can be given on symptomatic grounds rather than bacteriological.

To sum-up: never repeat the homoeopathic remedy as long as improvement continues. When improvement stops repeat the remedy in the same potency and if improvement does not follow give a higher potency, because we know, although it cannot yet be fully explained, that higher potencies maintain their effects for a longer time. In a patient who is undoubtedly recovering it is unnecessary to prescribe for aches and pains which he may complain of as these will disappear when full recovery has taken place, and one never wants to multiply remedies. However it does sometimes occur that a patient complains of some inter-current symptom like severe neuralgia which is obviously not responding to the main remedy although the general condition is so much better. Then it is quite justifiable to give an intercurrent remedy to relieve it. This however must be chosen from similarity to the particular symptoms in question and will probably be related to the main remedy (as *Aconite* is to *Sulphur*) in its curative properties. This remedy should be given in a low potency if it has to be given at all. In that case the main high potency will go on working. It is necessary to review the case in its entirety from time to time as changes may possibly occur in the symptom-complex which will call for a new remedy.

It is a curious and interesting experience that while recovery is taking place symptoms of old or even forgotten troubles may recur. This does not mean that a new remedy is required. It bears out a fact which is frequently observed, that symptoms are cured in the reverse order of their appearance. The last shown is the first to clear. The other directions of cure noted by the homoeopaths are from within out and from above downward.

8

Childhood to Old Age

When I started in practice I found that a large number of patients possessed a little leather-bound case containing ten or twelve simple homoeopathic remedies. These had been handed down from their parents or grandparents and usually included a short list of instructions quoted from Dr Skinner, or some other homoeopathic doctor.

One that was always present was *Chamomilla*. This is a wonderful remedy for teething troubles, of every kind.

I remember a young couple who were worn out by their baby's screams, and who finally asked if anything could be done by homoeopathy. The child was given *Chamomilla* 30 nightly for a week and from the first night he gave no more trouble.

The same thing happened two or three years later with their second baby, and the mother suggested asking for more of the homoeopathic medicine. But the father by this time thought that the earlier improvement had been just chance and would have occurred anyhow, and was, therefore, against having more; so the household suffered night after night until the mother got in touch with a homoeopath and asked for help. Again *Chamomilla* 30 was given and there was complete restoration of peace in the household after the first night.

Another childhood complaint which we frequently tackle is car-sickness. For this there may be several remedies to choose from, but, unless there are contra-indications in the way of a very marked history of other complaints associated with the child's story, *Cocculus indicus* 30 is a most useful and rewarding medicine. There was once, as an example, a child of eighteen months who was brought to see her greatgrandmother for the first time. The poor child arrived looking very pale and wan and sobbing whenever she was spoken to. And this at the very moment when the young parents wanted her to make a very good impression. The greatgrandmother gave her one dose of *Cocculus* 30, and a few doses for the parents to take away with them. Subsequently the child was given a dose of this remedy before a long drive after which she became a perfectly normal traveller.

Cocculus 30 is also most useful for sea-sickness both for children and adults. A tablet of this was once given to a small boy who became more and more pea-green during a stormy crossing of the Bay of Biscay. Half an hour later he was rushing round the deck, and when asked how he felt he replied 'Oh it's quite calm now!'

Again this is a great remedy for air-sickness and I find that men rely upon it a lot. One man to whom it was given dreaded flying because he was apt to feel dizzy: several times he had actually fainted in the aircraft causing general panic. He still travels a great deal and when a journey lies ahead it is certain that whatever else he may forget to pack it would not be his *Cocculus*.

Another complaint for which homoeopathic medicine is very efficacious is bed-wetting (enuresis). Children who suffer from it often are very sensitive about it. There was spectacular improvement in a boy at a prep. school after a nightly dose of *Pulsatilla*. The Matron immediately asked if she could have a large bottle of these pills for her to use in the school, having previously obtained the parents' permission. And until she retired it was one of her medical mainstays. *Pulsatilla* is not the only remedy by any means. Involuntary escape of urine both during the day and night which necessitates the frequent change of clothing and bedclothes, is efficaciously controlled by *Natrum muriaticum*. Where incontinence has been controlled by this remedy the patient is found to have a great desire for salt and the typically mapped tongue as well as the frequently seen crack in the middle of the lower lip, which are so often symptomatic prescribing factors in giving this drug.

Sulphur is another remedy for enuresis which can be very useful.

It is most effective for the lean, pale child who loves sugar, fat and highly seasoned food, and yet is always hungry, generally abhors being washed and often sleeps with his feet out of bed.

Two other remedies are also invaluable in treating enuresis: first is *Causticum*. One of the characteristic symptoms indicating its use is weakness and spasms in various parts of the body, especially in the neck. Urine may spurt whenever the patient coughs. In children this remedy for bed-wetting has a very definite history. It is that the incontinence almost always occurs in the first sleep. The child is also worse in dry, clear, fine weather, always better in wet weather. This is one of the most marked of the *Causticum* symptoms, whatever the complaint for which it is used. *Thuja* also is invaluable when the child has to get up frequently lest the bed be saturated. Incidentally bed wetting symptoms needing this remedy may follow or be greatly increased by a bad reaction to vaccination.

Now I want to mention chilblains—I always feel that orthodox medicine rather neglects or ignores this condition, whereas in homoeopathy there is much that can be done. One can treat the immediate conditions with medicines covering the pathology only, or one can give patients the constitutional remedy which will so often give a permanent cure and improve the whole circulation. Among the remedies acting locally the most useful are *Agaricus*, *Secale* and *Tamus communis*. In the provings of *Secale* for instance, the circulation was very often drastically affected. There was a time when perfectly healthy fingers and toes became gangrenous as a result of eating rye infected with ergot mould (*Secale*). The proving of *Secale* was done before this cause of gangrene was identified, so it was being used homoeopathically before there was any knowledge of the source of the condition. This is another confirmation of the homoeopathic principle that likes should be treated by likes.

Agaricus is a remedy for acute sensitiveness to cold and damp when the patient frequently complains of itching and a redness and a burning sensation in the hands and feet. It is a remedy which was constantly used in the winter, although now not so often since centrally-heated houses are more common.

Tamus communis which is made from black bryony, can be used as a paint on the areas affected by chilblains, and quickly removes pain and gives great relief.

Infantile eczema is another complaint that responds well to homoeopathy. There was a small and very intelligent little boy of seventeen months who had severe eczema on his face, neck and feet and hands. For the first few weeks he did not respond to the homoeopathic remedies such as *Petroleum* or *Sulphur* that had been tried, but when given *Graphites* 6 in tablet form he improved within a very short time. This remedy is essentially a trituration of prepared black lead. His skin is now perfectly clear.

An unusually severe case was one in which a girl of ten was brought to see if homoeopathy would do her any good. The hands were extremely sore, cracked and bleeding and often oozing a thick yellow discharge. The patient went to school daily with both thumbs and three fingers of each hand bound up. Consequently she found great difficulty in writing and doing her work. She had been to see two skin specialists in the country but had got no better with any treatment whether ointments or local applications of heat rays. *Graphites* 6 was prescribed and the dermatologist was told by letter that she had been given a homoeopathic medicine made from lead. He wrote back to say that he had never heard of lead being given for skin complaints but he would wait to see what happened. Within a few weeks her hands and fingers were clear and only one thumb was giving trouble. This had since cleared up.

A tendency to colds and catarrh is commonly met with in childhood and the symptoms are usually covered by the patients' constitutional remedy. Where there is a marked family history of tuberculosis or chest infections, *Medorrhinum* and *Tuberculinum* are most useful. When no other symptoms or signs are present the snuffly baby responds very well to *Calcarea lactate*. For childhood catarrh *Pulsatilla* must be also mentioned: it is one of our homoeopathic 'sheet-anchors'. It is often needed most when accompanied by a frequent and persistent discharge of a thick yellow catarrh. The patient finds great relief in the open air but upon entering a room, particularly a hot room, all the symptoms reappear. At night the child's nose gets greatly stuffed up and this is followed by a copious flow in the morning; however, upon rising they feel better for moving about. These children are often weepy and crave sympathy and fussing. Catarrh accompanied by bronchial coughs responds to such remedies as *Ipecacuanha*, the infants' friend, which is unequalled in its usefulness for infantile bronchitis. This acute illness usually starts suddenly;·the child suffers from a suffocating cough and gags with a rattling that can be heard all over the room. The cough may be spasmodic accompanied by nausea and vomiting, and is eventually cleared by the *Ipecacuanha*. If it does not clear quickly *Antimonium tartaricum* might be needed, particularly if the child must be sat up to relieve his breathing, and has an accumulation of mucus in the chest which is thick, white and very difficult to clear. He looks sunken and sickly and often has a bluish face and is covered with cold sweat. It is frequently noticed that the child who needs *Calcarea carbonica* is very susceptible to the first cold spell. It is a common thing for a mother to say, 'She's not ill but her catarrh has started after catching a bad cold, and unless it is stopped now it will go on all winter'. If the child is a fat, flabby type, and if upon asking more about her history, her mother says that she is generally rather slow and does not keep up well with other children of her age, this remedy is particularly efficient.

There was the case of a little girl of ten who was doing very badly at school and was altogether rather miserable. She had a teacher who was always telling her she could do better, or that she did not try hard enough, and she would often arrive home in tears. She was a great worrier; she fretted over her work, about anyone who was ill in the street where she lived, or some injustice that she had seen. Weeping she would tell her family about it and probably repeat it several times. Her elder sister refused to sleep in the same room because she talked to herself about all her troubles and some nights awoke screaming from nightmares, and then would describe these to anyone who would listen. She had a large face and was very pale, and looked as if she had no go. She was given *Calcarea carbonica* 10m. and did not need to return to the doctor for a year. By then she had skipped a form and was second in her school examinations. She is now grown up and has done very well in her work and life. When she is worried or is not sleeping well this patient asks for a few powders of *Calc. carb.* usually about once a year.

Acne—this is one of the more common complaints of adolescence and there are many difficult cases which we as homoeopaths see. In very recent years tetracycline has been frequently administered for long spells but as yet we do not really know enough about its long-term side effects. Although the patient's skin can improve on the antibiotic for as long as he continues to take it, his disposition often deteriorates and he can suffer depression as well as loss of weight and appetite. We have found that as soon as the treatment stops the complaint generally reappears. What is more, many adolescents do not respond to the antibiotic and these are those whom homoeopathy greatly helps. The skin specialists recognize the difficulty of treating this condition; where there has been a family incidence it usually lasts the same number of years in each generation, and can be controlled by tetracycline when it is bad. However, there is so much that the homoeopathic doctor can do with his good, commonsense medicine in treating the patient and relieving the ailment and its causes, whereas any treatment for a superficial problem risks doing other damage which may be transient or permanent, but which can be a greater hazard than the condition from which the patient suffers. One can say that any symptom of disorder or disease surely reflects one fact, namely, that in that individual there is disease or disorder and this is general and not confined to a particular organ or tissue.

Every week our consulting room is visited by doctors who are anxious to learn about homoeopathy. At a morning session when four doctors were present, we saw an eighteen year old girl suffering from the worst possible outbreak of acne. She gave us her background. Her parents had been separated and the skin trouble started four years ago after her mother's death and her father did not want her back. In fact nobody wanted her. An uncle said he would pay to equip her for a job but again she felt that he would want to be finished with her. She told us she was worried about her future and that her moods varied from hour to hour and that she was extremely constipated. *Natrum muriaticum* was prescribed in high potency and she was told to come back in a fortnight. When she did so one barely recognized the pretty bright girl who walked in with her face practically clear—she was only seen once more, but after a year she sent a request for more medicine. Her skin had been perfectly all right but she had been very worried over her first job, and she thought it might start again although it had not so far!

Adolescent behaviour problems can respond extremely well to homoeopathy. One so often sees the restless, dissatisfied teenager who wants change and excitement, and for whom nothing can ever be right, and who, in consequence upsets the whole household. The girl who cannot concentrate on her work, and if she crams the week before her exams may get a very bad headache. There is the boy who never stops blaming the school to which he was sent, or the people he has to meet, and who is unwilling to take a share in entertaining friends, who hates talking to people and wants to wander about and do what he likes. If given *Calcarea phosphoricum* at this stage these youngsters become different personalities and are probably saved from starting to take drugs at a later stage.

There was a typical case of alopoecia in a lad of eighteen who came to see if we could do anything to grow his hair.

He was completely bald, without eyebrows or eyelashes. He gave his general history and in the course of doing so told us there was no history of baldness in his family. He had some indigestion and said that although he got very hungry he did not have a large appetite. He worried his mother by pushing away his plate after only a few mouthfuls, yet he loved sweet things and could be persuaded to eat more if he was given jam with his meat. If he were left alone in a room with a box of chocolates he would certainly finish the box—he was nervous and apprehensive and not really a good mixer. This is the kind of case where *Lycopodium* works most effectively. A month later he appeared with a little mat of hair over his head and his eyebrows, and eyelashes had started to grow.

A number of cases of alopoecia occur in teenagers and they usually have been told when they go to see a doctor about it that there was nothing to be done. Homoeopathy does not achieve successes in every case, but in a large proportion of cases where this treatment is used good results have been obtained.

In treating conditions of stiffness or injuries in the teenager the homoeopathic doctor has at hand that wonderful remedy *Arnica*, which is made from *Arnica montana*. Every good homoeopath probably has a supply of it. A friend was most interested and surprised because she had seen the name *Arnica* on her mother's medicine. She had just returned from climbing in Switzerland and learned that many of the Swiss guides chewed Arnica leaves when doing their first climb of the year. They used it, they said, because it stopped them from being stiff afterwards. A teenage schoolboy who was captain of his football team heard of this and took a bottle with him to use at school. There was soon a request for a large bottle. He had given it round the team, and none of them experienced stiffness after their first game and he wanted a supply to use when necessary. It is also the first and best remedy for any injury. It stops a great deal of the bruising and swelling and helps the patient to recover much more rapidly. A doctor at one of our Intensive Courses of homoeopathy said that he could not be more interested in this form of medicine but he was very busy and had not the time to study it and so what should he do? He was certainly intending to return for the next course so it was suggested that for the next three months he should try out *Arnica*— giving it for any bruising or injury—before and after an operation and even for exhaustion and fatigue. A letter arrived before the next Intensive Course asking if he could give a very quick ten minute talk on his results with *Arnica*— he found it such an astounding remedy.

I have found that surgeons like *Arnica* to be prescribed and always remember one who, whenever I attended an operation upon one of my patients, used to greet me with 'Blackie have you given *Arnica*?'

Anxiety is an emotion from which anyone may suffer to a greater or lesser extent. And we have found *Argentum nitricum* taken before examinations, speaking or public appearances affects a calming influence almost immediately. Some of the old homoeopaths used to call it 'the funk pills'. I heard of a man recently who wrote from Australia to ask for some of the homoeopathic 'funk pills'. He had two boys of eleven and twelve who were facing exams and he remembered the wonderful pills he had been given before his final exams in England when he was in his teens.

In adolescence and adult life migraine is one of the complaints which homoeopathy can help quite considerably. Taking two examples: one, the case of a schoolmaster who was quite desperate over the increasing frequency of his extreme migraine. He was the deputy headmaster and at the end of term had to interview all the other teachers in order to make a full term report. If he had migraine he could not face this. He described the headache as starting at the back of the neck and travelling up the head ending on the right temple, and if very bad he was apt to be sick with it. With onset of the headache he was inclined to sweat and got damp, and was painfully aware of his offensive smelling, sweating feet. He was always worse for a cold wind and at night used to wrap his head in a shawl and found that lying on a hot water bottle gave enormous relief. Because of his whole symptom picture he was given *Silica* in a high potency. He could hardly believe it when week after week went by without his getting a migraine—he had only the occasional very slight headache but nevertheless was able to do his work. He did not need a repeat of the *Silica* for a year when again it had a dramatic effect. After that it was learned that he never suffered from migraine again.

The second case is of a woman of forty who lives under continuous strain. Two or three times a month she wakes in the morning with a severe headache and her vision is affected so that she has zig zags of light in front of her eyes. She feels sick and very unwell, also the headache is always worse during menstruation, when it would possibly lift in the afternoon or go on into the next day. She has a great desire for salt and is unable to face a meal without taking far too much. On physical examination the only thing found was a slight rise in blood-pressure which rather frightened her as it ran in the family. In this case *Natrum muriaticum* was prescribed with rapid improvement as a result.

In adult life homoeopathy is again invaluable. The homoeopathic doctor meets a number of cases where a young business man has felt unduly tired and finds his work rather a burden or, worse still, feels that he is not grasping it as well as he did. To give one typical example, a tall, stooping and worried-looking young man came to try homoeopathy. When he got up in the morning, feeling a dread of the day ahead, he wondered if he could face it. By the time he had forced himself up and got to work, he was all right, but he was dead tired when he got home at about six in the evening and would just sit in a chair and hope not to be disturbed—he said that that was his worst time of the day. He would buck-up after that and if he were going out would thoroughly enjoy his evening. Then he found he was often slow in going to sleep, his mind being too active and not allowing him to relax.

He used to go to the country for most weekends, and his brother would make him play strenuous games of tennis or take long cross-country walks sometimes over heavy ploughed land. He was then so exhausted that he felt quite frightened and at that stage rather insecure and would worry as to whether he would be able to carry on with his work and if he had the stamina to tackle it. He had a small appetite but at times used to be hungry soon after a meal and would then eat sweets or chocolates to keep himself going. He always wanted his food very hot, complaining that cold food affected his digestion. He felt the cold weather but disliked a stuffy room. He did not want a lot of company but invariably preferred it if someone was within call, although he hardly liked confessing this fact. He took a long time to give his full history as he was temperamentally reticent and had been called haughty at school because he did not easily make friends. He did not sweat easily and said that he would be better if he did. He complained that recently he was forgetting names and sometimes left important words out of sentences. He was given *Lycopodium* in high potency and he was grateful for the subsequent feeling of well-being within a week or two.

Depression is one of the most difficult conditions, but if the patient can get homoeopathic remedies early there is no doubt that he will often recover without further treatment. A very depressed middle-aged woman visited a homoeopathic doctor accompanied by her sister (who was herself a patient) in case she failed to admit how depressed she really was. She had lost her husband and her younger son who had always lived at home with her was now about to be married. Further, he was being transferred to another department of his work which necessitated his moving away from her. She sat in a chair and hardly spoke a word while her sister explained all this—no effort to rouse her was at all successful, and it was hard to get even a word from her. This type of uncooperative patient responds well to *Aurum metallicum* which she was given and she was told to come again in a fortnight. When she came she was a different person, calm, answering any questions and very much better and she remained so. Recently she came once more—this time because she was getting a little depressed and the remedy was repeated with equally good effect.

Another case was in a young man who was extremely depressed and again did not want to talk about it. He had been like this on and off for two or three years and had an unfortunate background. He had felt burdened by a false sense of guilt over a family tragedy and this had resulted in skin eruptions which added to his depression. He had been in a mental home where he had been given shock treatment. He was very unhappy and could not talk to his family since he felt they did not understand him. He was given *Aurum metallicum* in a high potency and felt it did a great deal of good. For the next year he called on a homoeopathic doctor every week, sometimes oftener, and it was found that *Natrum muriaticum* 6 kept him going fairly well. Every now and then the high potency of *Aurum metallicum* was repeated with further improvement. He gradually became better and better and nowadays lives a perfectly normal life.

Firstly in the treatment of rheumatic complaints there is the patient with a general rheumatism which is aggravated by cold wet weather, who claims that because of his pains he knows when it is about to rain. The patient who describes his rheumatism as wandering from joint to joint, who says when one joint is relieved another is attacked with severe pain and whose rheumatism is generally worse in the summer and is often accompanied by painful shin-bones. He also finds that the rheumatism alternates with digestive troubles—all these symptoms will clear up with *Kali bichromicum.*

Then there is the rheumatic patient who is prone to backache or, indeed, pain anywhere who always, once again, seems to know when it is going to rain and feels worse in very cold, wet weather. This patient is often worse for sea bathing and from undue strain, and finds considerable relief from a hot bath or warm application. This is the patient who is very stiff on getting up in the morning but who limbers up after gentle exercise. His stiffness may return if he sits in a chair for too long and he may get up and walk about at night to ease his pain. He may be generally restless and must move about although it may be painful at first. For such cases *Rhus toxicodendron* in a high potency will probably give quick and lasting relief.

There is the rheumatic patient who needs *Pulsatilla* whose pains shift rapidly from part to part, and who is increasingly chilly with the pains but who is worse for heat; particularly in bed, and is relieved by uncovering and lying in cool open air. Also he is very sensitive to a sudden jar or pressure. This patient often has very changeable moods; can be irritable, then weeping, then smiling all within a few minutes. Pains will be described as drawing, tearing in the limbs and these are better for movement and remain better after motion, but the aches are again worse in a warm room, and respond well to cold applications on a joint.

Another invaluable rheumatic remedy that must be mentioned is *Bryonia*. When the rheumatism comes on in dry cold weather with acute pain and swelling around joints and which is worse for the slightest movement, such a patient wants to be quite still and not disturbed. He can get very irritable when questioned or talked to. The tongue here is coated white and he is intensely thirsty for long cold drinks—he is frequently constipated with dry hard stools. His pains are stitching in character and there is often violent local inflammation and the affected area is very hot. If he perspires he feels better. If the patient is running a temperature or if his rheumatic condition is very acute, he likes to keep quite still and will lie on the affected joint. He can also look dull and purplish, and become quite muddly when he is ill. He may then ask to 'go home' as he does not really know where he is. He may have an acute headache with his rheumatism but again buries his head in the pillow and does not move.

The final more common remedy for rheumatism to be mentioned here is *Nux vomica*. Some years ago a man used to get acute rheumatic pains—particularly in the lumbar region—he was much worse if he moved and complained that he had to sit up in order to turn round in the night. He had a dread of moving. He was extremely chilly, and could not bear to uncover. He repeatedly said how much better he felt after getting really warm and having a very hot drink. He used to be incredibly irritable and snappy when his rheumatism flared up. He reported the marked relief he had one day, which he said was due to the weather; it was a wet, muggy morning; everyone was surprised, but he claimed that it was so much better than the dry, cold weather which we had been having and he liked the rain! It had always suited him. This marked symptom confirmed the conviction that *Nux vomica* was what was needed.

To the orthodox doctor every case of shingles is the same, varying only in degree. To the homoeopathic doctor each patient reacts differently and is prescribed for on that particular reaction. The first case is of a woman with a very bad early patch of shingles on the right side of her head. It was already spreading up into the head and down to her eyebrow and eyelid on that side and was intensely painful. She could not stand a draught or cold of any kind and she felt better if she held hot lint to the affected areas. She was very restless and found herself getting up to move about every few minutes. She even thought that she felt better after moving. She was given *Rhus toxicodendron*; it checked further spread and was healing well a few days later when seen again.

An American woman came in with a vesicular rash on her arm. 'If I'd been at home' she said 'I'd have thought I'd been in a poison ivy bush—it gives that kind of rash.' In its provings Poison Ivy (*Rhus toxicodendron*) produced just such vesicular rashes and many other symptoms— all these symptoms of a patient needing *Rhus tox.* are the better for heat, worse for resting and beginning to move but relieved by continued movement.

There are a number of other homoeopathic remedies that can help in the case of shingles. When the sufferer is worse for heat and on the contrary likes cool air to the rash, *Ranunculus bulbosus* (buttercup) is the remedy which is indicated. If the shingles is swollen and purplish around the rash and the patient longs for cold application, then *Lachesis* (snake venom) should be given. In these cases the left side is most often affected. If its progress is slow and the shingles are not clearing then *Variolinum* may be needed.

More people suffer from piles than wish to confess to it. *Aesculus hippocastanum* (horse chestnut) has been proved to be a great pile remedy with a definite symptom picture. As a rule the haemorrhoids are blind but if they bleed it gives relief. There is a constant sensation of dryness, fullness and pricking in the rectum as if little sticks or splinters were pricking the folds of mucous membrane, often accompanied by a weak, stiff sensation in the lower back as if the legs would give way. As a rule the patient is constipated with large stools which are very hard and followed by a feeling of prolapse of the rectum accompanied by backache. The patient feels that he can't stand and finds walking difficult.

Nitric acid is another remedy that we find very useful, particularly when the piles bleed after every evacuation. These patients are apt to have a fissure and then get a spasm of the anus with splinter-like pain and a continued urging to stool which comes with much bleeding. The haemorrhoids also protrude very often when they bleed, and the rectum often feels that it is torn asunder during a stool. This is as a rule a cold, thin, dark patient who is usually of a melancholy disposition and who has a deep fear about his health. He can be bad tempered and fly into a rage and may then be inclined to weep; but he is often very despairing and this covers his general unfitness. He is also very obstinate. He is one of the chilly, fat loving people although fat upsets him.

Ruta graveolens (rue); this remedy has had a great repute in medicine over many years for epilepsy, hysteria, weakness of sight, piles and inertia of bowels with very difficult stools. It is often most useful when piles are starting and we have met a great many patients where the symptoms have cleared completely, and even where prolapse of the rectum has never occurred again.

Ratanhia is the root of several species of Krameria, and

this again is a remedy of long standing repute. It is in all its species intensely astringent. The symptoms are those of great straining and resulting in a very hard stool so that the patient can cry out when it passes. There is commonly a profusion of piles and the burning sensation lasts for a long time after the evacuation. Even if the stool is loose this burning still persists and is characteristic. There are one or two strange and peculiar symptoms associated with *Ratanhia*. The molar teeth feel as if cold rushes out of them and there are sensations as if the rectum was all twisted up or as if splinters of glass were in the rectum, as if the rectum protruded and then went back with a jerk. Some of the old homoeopathic doctors thought that this remedy covered more rectal symptoms than any other.

The remedy *Sulphur* has many rectal symptoms in its drug picture and with its other troubles piles are a common complaint. These protrude, ooze and bleed. The anus becomes very much inflamed and swollen and is some-times excoriated with a lot of irritation all round and often oozing from the rectum. Then *Sulphur* will fit the patient with these definite local symptoms, together with the stooping hot-blooded, untidy characteristics of this drug which have already been described.

Causticum can also be a great constitutional remedy for a patient suffering from piles which impede the stool and which are stinging and burning and worse from touch or washing, and where there is frequently a fissure present. This is needed in the chilly patient with a tendency to contractions of muscles who becomes very worried in the evening because of anxious thoughts, and is often peevish and irritable because he thinks something awful is impend-ing. He is very apt to have weak and irritated eyes, as if sand were in them and the patient either wants to shut his eyes or they close involuntarily and he feels he cannot open them. His eyes pour tears in the open air.

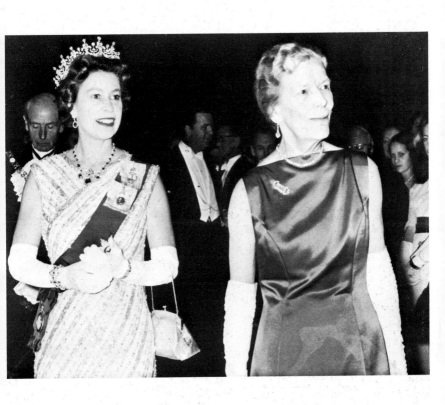

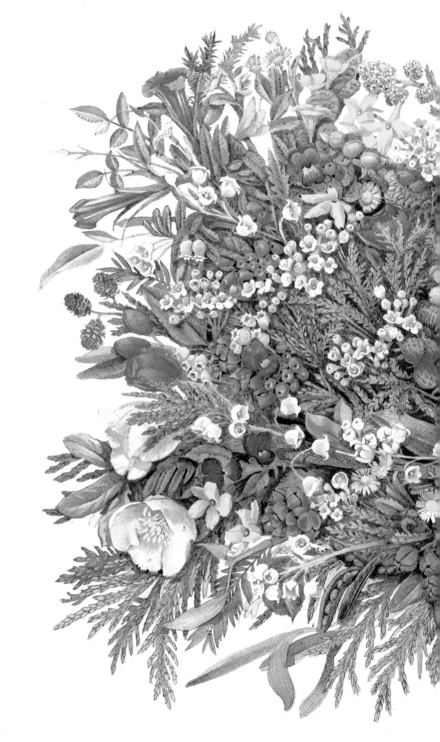

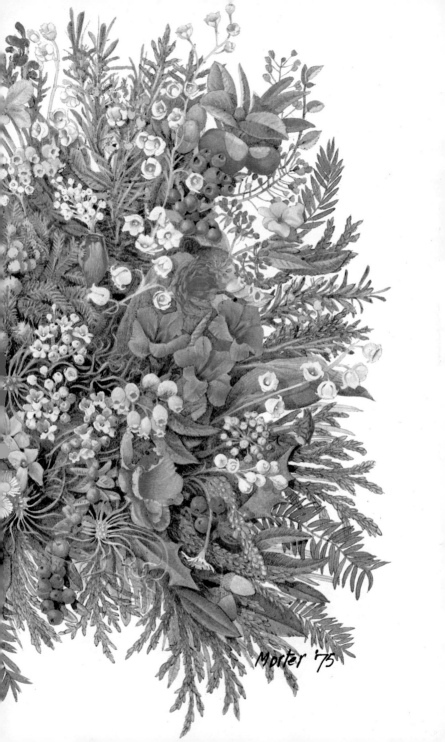
Morter '75

Black and white photograph

Her Majesty Queen Elizabeth II and Dr Margery Blackie (by Gracious Permission of Her Majesty The Queen). Taken at a Homoeopathic Reception held at The Guildhall on 20th October 1970, when forty-three homoeopathic doctors were presented to Her Majesty.

Colour plate

A painting of the programme-holder bouquet presented to Her Majesty The Queen on the occasion of her visit to the Royal London Homoeopathic Hospital, of which she is a patron. The forty-two flowers, plants and seeds represent some of the natural sources of homoeopathic medicines readily found in almost every part of the world.

This is the patient who may get facial paralysis in a cold wind, is ravenously hungry and eats very fast but his appetite goes quickly. It is one of the best bladder remedies and is often characterized by an urging to urinate and he cannot pass water but it may then escape involuntarily while he is sitting, or if he coughs or sneezes.

Loss of voice and hoarseness are often helped by *Causticum*. This is most effective for someone who gets a stiffness in the back and neck in a cold wind or whose condition improves markedly when it rains. It is also characteristic that this person may have an eruption of pimples on the nose, an itching moist patch on the neck and general itching all over.

Menopausal difficulties also respond extremely well to homoeopathic remedies and one of the remedies most needed in *Sepia*. This is made from the famous liquid contained in the ink-bag of the cuttle fish. There are two types who may need this wonderful medicine. The first is the definitely indignant woman who won't come of her own accord but is persuaded or even driven to come and resents the fact that she is unwell; or the definitely dull and stupid looking woman who may be stubborn but is more often just over-tired, with a slow acting brain. The patient has a fatter face than one would expect from the rest of her build, and the sallow yellow colour is not met with in any other drug. She has dark rings under her eyes spreading half way down her cheeks and often there is a characteristic brownish saddle across her nose. She usually has warts on her neck and face which go brownish later on in life. Her lips are pale and she has to make an obvious effort to hold up her long back.

She has a general resentment against fate and thinks she has had a poor deal. If you console her she will probably round on you as she hates sympathy; but if her defences break down on telling her story she may weep and, if she does, always feels much better afterwards.

She is the tired out patient—nervously, mentally and physically. She appears dull and may weep a lot once she has started and she says she feels beaten and cannot go on. If the doctor sets out to cheer her he is met by an obstinate disagreeable resentful mood, and in this state she feels a martyr. People are not fair to her and she does not want to be interfered with and she may become melancholic, hopeless and taciturn and doesn't want to be either helped or made well.

This is her characteristic picture but under great stress she may become more excitable and very restless. If a neighbour offers help she will get snapped at. It is more than the patient can stand, and she has a great fear of something more dreadful happening. Her children are going to be ill—her husband isn't well and they will all be homeless and she dreads poverty—she has always been independent and she would hate to ask for help—she can become envious of others who haven't her difficulties and can be very spiteful in her remarks. The patient needing *Sepia* is worse in a stuffy room which can make her feel faint, and she can very easily faint on standing or on kneeling in church. On the whole this woman is chilly and doesn't stand the cold or damp well and she is worse in changes of weather particularly when changing from dry to damp. She is worse in the morning unless she has had a sleep. She gets a dragging sensation in the pelvis and feels full there. Her menstrual periods are scanty or irregular and often painful. She complains of backache which improves as she walks about but on first rising is very painful and better for pressure from a cushion at her back on sitting.

All *Sepia* patients have certain marked symptoms. They are better for movement and can often walk or dance themselves well. They are all relieved by sleep—all are improved with food. They complain of palpitation with a sensation that the heart will force its way through the chest wall. Walking fast will take it off. Finally it is a very useful medicine in sterility.

Here again one must mention *Pulsatilla* for the patient who is very troubled by hot flushes which wake her several times at night and are very frequent in the day and worse in a hot airless room. She then often suffers from lack of sleep and goes over and over things in the night. Her tongue looks normal although it feels dry and in spite of this she is thirstless. She is apt to get pains everywhere with her change of life. These are often rheumatic and move from place to place and, like most pains in a patient needing *Pulsatilla*, always characteristically come suddenly and go gradually. These pains are better for gentle movement and the patient often says that she gets up at night to move about and perhaps make a warm drink and sleeps so much better after. The pain is worse if she bandages a joint.

She has usually been the plump loving child, and during adolescence has frequently been spoilt by the rest of the family because she is so pretty and likes fuss, so that in middle age she may be rather selfish and demanding. She still hates to be alone and loves company and can burst into tears very easily but can usually be quickly cheered up. This patient always complains of the heat and hot weather and cannot sit directly in the sun. She likes to move about gently in the open air. She hates fatty food as it upsets her and is often followed by nausea, vertigo and headache, a headache which is worse on stooping.

Quite often this patient will sleep with her arms above her head.

Squid like *Sepia* is one of the sea remedies and was differentiated from *Sepia* by Dr W. E. Boyd of Glasgow and

Dr Stearns of USA. Both said it was not synonymous with *Sepia* and although squids are cuttle fish, preparation was not made from fresh 'ink' only.

This remedy is often needed by most normal people at the menopause—frequently they are energetic, quick and intelligent, very hard workers. Of all the women treated by the sea remedies they are the most genuinely interested in other people, and are the least self-centered of this group, unlike the irritable, tired martyred *Sepia* patient.

She is rather sleepless before menstruation and often has quite severe mastitis the week before. She is very chilly and she herself finds work more of an effort, but the only thing noticeable is that anyone who works with her has to jump to it. She is impatient, not irritable. One usually wonders if one will give *Sepia* because of the depression, but the picture is really quite different here, not the same degree of backache or irritability. This remedy is really only needed at the menopause. The whole group of the sea remedies is particularly useful then, but *Squid* is probably needed only at that time.

In writing about homoeopathy one must also mention the neurotic patient who is given tranquillizers, probably sleeping pills, and sometimes even anti-depressants for treatment. As a rule these patients have no actual disease and are not really ill but they find it very difficult to live a normal life and are often afraid of tackling a job. They come to the doctor with a great many symptoms which they like to describe fully but which quite often mean very little. It is not at all easy to deal with them, but through the years patients have been given their constitutional remedy and it has helped considerably. In these cases one likes to use a high potency and see how much it will do. But there are often so many complaints that it is justifiable to give a low potency of a remedy like *Coffea* or *Lycopodium* to help the sleeplessness; or *Argentum nitricum* to the patient who dares not go shopping alone and may become panicky if she feels closed in. *Aurum* 6 can be useful if they are depressed or they may be greatly helped by *Natrum muriaticum* 6 if they feel rather resentful that life has not treated them better.

It is very satisfactory to find them taking the risk of doing a job and both doing it well and enjoying it. This is another instance of where homoeopathy can help a patient to make more of an effort and if possible get on with life without being under the influence of drugs which may produce sleepiness or prevent clear thinking.

Head injuries treated by homoeopathy frequently respond very well. A man in his early 60s was involved in a motor accident. On X-ray examination no fracture was found but he complained of continuous headache which varied in severity and was worse if he had to concentrate or spend time doing paper work, and worse if he had to travel, which was part of his job. He also complained that he had troublesome catarrh all the time since the accident and he was extremely worried and depressed. He was given *Arnica* first but, although the patient felt better in himself, his headache was the same. He was then given *Natrum sulph*, one of the best of the after-injury remedies, and he began to improve at once and within a week or two felt completely well again. He has had no return of headache or catarrh.

A recent case had very severe head pains after a head injury. She was very dull and heavy looking and was given *Opium* with considerable help. In homoeopathic use *Opium* is a frequently used medicine for injury with these symptoms. It is also one of the standbys for shock and for strokes—in each of which there is semi-consciousness or dullness and inability to concentrate. This patient, however, did not completely clear up on *Opium* and was given *Cicuta* because she became very nervously irritable and very annoyed with herself. She is doing very well.

The third case I would like to mention was a girl who again was involved in an accident and on X-ray was found to have a fractured skull. She had a severe headache after but was seen by a neurologist and surgeon who both advised doing nothing as there was no pressure from the fracture. She was given *Natrum sulph* with steady relief and has never had any symptoms since.

Homoeopathic remedies frequently prove their efficacy in helping those who have suffered a stroke or shock. Their effectiveness is best illustrated by giving an example: A retired colonel, in his early 60s, ran a big estate in the country when his agent suddenly fell ill. This put an unaccustomed burden on the owner who found that he had to do more paper work and more supervising of the actual day-to-day running of the estate. He himself at this time was in delicate health having been treated homoeopathically for Buergers disease and other illnesses. One day he came into the house with a very red face complaining of a severe headache, and very soon thereafter he lost consciousness. His wife immediately rang his GP and his homoeopathic doctor. The GP got in touch with a consultant and later that day all three were at the patient's bedside. The consultant examined the man and found his blood pressure very high indeed; with that and his deep unconsciousness he diagnosed a 'cerebral catastrophe' and thought he would not live. He gave the nurse who was present various instructions and then asked if the homoeopathic doctor had any suggestions. This doctor said that if he were prescribing he would put a powder of *Opium* (high potency) on to his tongue. 'Oh,' the consultant exclaimed, 'how pleased my mother would have been! She was such a great homoeopath.' The unconscious man was given the powders and the doctors left. Three hours later, just as the nurse was getting ready for the night, a voice from the bed said, 'What about dinner?' From that moment on the patient made a steady improvement. He recovered completely and for the next ten years lived a normal life running his estate and remained one of the best shots in the county.

Many examples could be given of the very beneficial effects of homoeopathic *Opium* for strokes. It is also a great remedy for patients in shock, especially those who have a history of having never felt the same since some family tragedy or shock. There was the case of the woman who was having coffee in a town on the coast with her brother and sister-in-law, both over eighty years of age when a bomb fell outside the restaurant and shattered all the glass. For the next two hours the patient hunted for her relations and couldn't find them anywhere. Finally, a policeman begged her to go home, promising to get in touch with her when he had news. She agreed and when she got home she found the old couple sitting in the garden! For several weeks she felt very unwell and muddleheaded. She then saw her homoeopathic doctor and as he dated all her symptoms back to this bomb incident he gave her a high potency of *Opium* and she was quite her old self within a few days.

A woman of seventy had a nervous breakdown and was given six shock treatments within a fortnight. She had had a wonderful life, had done excellent social work, and was greatly loved and respected. She always liked homoeopathy and asked to be treated by it whenever possible, so after the shock therapy she had her homoeopathic treatment steadily for six months. At the end of that time the homoeopathic doctor called to see her and found her surrounded by books and preparing to translate English and French books, a job in which she was greatly interested.

She was an expert at this and greatly enjoyed the work it entailed. She carried on with her translating for several years, and if she was overtired used to take a few doses of *Arnica* 6 which she kept by her, or of *Lycopodium* 6, which was her constitutional remedy three times a day for a week. She said it always did her good and helped her memory. When she was getting on for eighty she had to have some-one living with her as she could not be left alone, or she might go out and forget where she lived or how to get home and she could, at that time, be very difficult.

Symptomatically, as in such cases, she would sometimes close her mouth tightly, refusing to speak, sometimes even to eat. She also had very changeable moods and at one time would read aloud for hours upon end—always from the same page. At another she would sing for hours, often at night. She was frequently inclined to be suspicious and would then refuse to take any medicine, and in a general way she was usually worse after sleep. She had had a lot of eye trouble and operations, but fortunately she could see to read almost to the end. She was obsessed by her fear of water and always had a very dry mouth. One night she refused to get into bed in spite of all the efforts by the nurse to make her do so; however she got in when her homoeo-pathic doctor arrived. Two of the homoeopaths then studied her case and sent *Hyoscyamus* 30 then 12, which kept her on an even keel for the rest of her life. She died peacefully in a nursing home where the nurses were most understanding and reassuring.

How satisfactory it is to treat a patient with these safe remedies which stimulate their own recuperative powers and which can be given in times of stress without fear of a bad reaction!

An old lady of eighty-three decided to have a hip

operation. She was given a few doses of *Arnica* beforehand, but the rest of her treatment was left to the surgical staff. She was very sleepless and no sedatives seemed to help. She became very wandering in her mind and kept the other patients awake with her incessant talking. Her daughter was terrified that she would never again regain normality. However, eventually she was well and she returned home. In six months she wrote to say that arthritic changes were progressing in the other hip and that she felt that they would increase. She might as well have both sides better. The surgeon was consulted in order to discuss the possibility of a second operation and the after treatment. He said that he would agree to her having exclusively homoeopathic remedies without any antibiotics or sleeping draughts. This time she had *Arnica* more frequently over the first forty-eight hours without any other dosing and she was perfectly calm and sensible all through her convalescence. She can now walk comfortably and carry out all she wants to do.

A third old lady had been treated for years by homoeopathy. She had had a very interesting life and had been president of a club for several years where she was extremely popular. She was difficult in that she would go abroad with her husband and go in for some treatment which they both fancied, so that they were apt to return with injections to be given, pills to take and many suggestions. However they always asked to return to homoeopathy within a week or two! After her husband's death at the age of eighty-five she was not so well and became very depressed. She was sure she was getting some dire disease—she did not want to see people and when they called she would often refuse to open her front door. She was given a high potency of *Sepia* as it fitted her moods and depression so well. It lifted her spirits markedly. She was by then rather weak and feeble and was given

Arsenicum when she complained of the cold and was full of fears, and *Arnica* when she felt exhausted, but these were given in the 6th potency so as to leave the high potency of *Sepia* working as it will go on doing for some months and with these remedies to help she died very peacefully.

I want to end this chapter with a brief mention of the hopeless cases that can be so helped by homoeopathy.

A man who was a florist took a great interest in homoeopathy and over many years had acquired a considerable knowledge of it, so much so that when he went to the flower market he always carried twelve little bottles of homoeopathic medicines in his waistcoat pockets. On arrival at the market he was often accosted with ' 'Guv'— have you anything for my skin—my hands are raw and cracking since I have had to handle such and such a plant'. The friend was given half a dozen tablets in an envelope to take four-hourly and how often they helped! When this man became very thin he was persuaded to see a doctor. He was sent to hospital for X-rays and investigation, was found to have a carcinoma of the stomach. An operation was suggested but was met by a firm refusal and the remark that 'something had to put him in the long box', he knew that homoeopathy would keep him going as well and as long as possible. He lived for about two years and used to get remarkable relief from gastric pains with the use of *Graphites* and *Carbo. vegetabilis* which relieved his wind and distension, and one of Dr Tyler's favourite remedies, a tincture of *Ornithogalum* (Star of Bethlehem) after food. Only in the last few days of his life did he have to have morphia. So hopeless cases can respond to this type of treatment and most patients are happier not having to feel half doped all the time in their last illness.

9

Homoeopathy in Ear, Nose and Throat Cases

There are more and more dentists, in the USA particularly, becoming interested in the homoeopathic treatment of mouth problems. Many patients present signs and symptoms in the mouth with which we are all familiar. Unhealthy gums have already been mentioned, but the incalculable help that can be given by *Calendula* mouth washes, and remedies such as one of the *Mercury* preparations, is being recognized more widely. The tincture of *Plantago* can give much marked relief from pain in a tooth. It is applied locally to the very sore area. Also *Lycopodium* taken as tablets is constantly found to be very good for toothache.

Silica is another remedy that can be invaluable, particularly in a tooth abscess and can even push out a diseased tooth. Then the condition of loose teeth which is commonly met with can be helped. *Calendula* comes in here again. A patient who will gently massage the gums towards the teeth and then hold a warm *Calendula* mouthwash which is a cleanser, in the mouth, will find the teeth tightening up and the condition much improved. Usually this is made more effective in combination with one of the *Calcium salts* as a remedy.

Aphthous ulcers are a subject on their own and have been fully discussed and investigated. Perhaps the most commonly needed remedies here are *Argentum nitricum* and *Thuja*, taking all their general symptoms into account when prescribing. The help of dentists has added to the understanding of these complaints in relation to the constitution of the patients. Local treatment has been found to be of little value but good results have been obtained by homoeopathy and are constantly being confirmed. It has been found, interestingly enough, that some of the best results have been obtained by giving of the patients constitutional remedy even where it did not produce aphthous ulcers in its *materia medica* provings. This confirms what every homoeopathic doctor knows that the nearer he can get to the patient's whole picture the better are the results.

There ought to be closer co-operation between dentists and patients' doctors in identifying the constitutional drug.

Another complaint in which homoeopathy may help is a cyst in the jaw. A boy of thirteen began to get a swelling inside his left cheek. It was somewhat painful and began to enlarge more and more and he was taken by a homoeopathic doctor to see an Ear, Nose and Throat specialist. Several X-rays were done and it was diagnosed as a cyst in the jawbone and an operation was advised. This was carried out five years ago and the patient was left with quite extensive swelling still on his left cheek. He was treated with *Symphytum* (made from comfrey) and gradually the swelling subsided and now it is practically normal. There has been no recurrence, which the surgeon warned might happen.

Some of the Ear, Nose and Throat surgeons are very

happy to have patients given *Arnica* before and after their operations. They confirm that it 'hurries healing, prevents bruising' and several have affirmed that it is useful in their opinion in preventing a recurrence of polypi.

A young woman who worked in South Africa had an enormous polypus removed from her nose. It was so big that it would hardly come through the nostril. On pathological examination it was found to be schwannoma which both the surgeon and pathologist thought might recur. She returned to South Africa after being given first *Arnica* and then *Calcarea phosphorica* to go on with. Two years later she was given special leave to see the surgeon again. He found everything perfectly normal and no sign of any recurrence. Since then she has reported regularly and has had one of the *Calcium salts* when needed.

Then in cases of sinusitis where the surgeon would normally feel inclined to drain the sinus and where, indeed, it has been done for previous attacks, it has been found frequently that homoeopathic remedies such as *Potassium salts* and *Silica*, particularly, have so helped the condition that nothing further is needed.

Otitis media, infection of middle ear, and other ear conditions can also be very much helped homoeopathically. As in cases of 'sticky ear', where the patient has had antibiotics in the acute phase, but which has not cleared the condition. The patient has come to consult a homoeopath to avoid having to have gromwetts put in to help drainage. With the advancing understanding of the chemistry of this problem of the discharge which collects and cannot drain, medical means of making it more liquid are very possible and even if homoeopathy was not used in the early stages it is found very useful later on. Homoeopathic *Mercury* has been quoted as the medical 'surgeon' for the middle ear.

Oto-sclerosis and Menière's disease, can be helped in very early stages and delay the need for an operation. This and tinnitus, noises in ears, are known to respond to homoeopathy and save the patients from surgical interference which does not always succeed. Some early operations done for the deafness caused by oto-sclerosis were performed in the Glasgow Homoeopathic Hospital and these patients were looked after by the homoeopathic physicians afterwards and the results were very good.

No one knows yet why tinnitus is associated with oto-sclerosis nor what makes one operation a success and another a failure in the relief of this very troublesome symptom. There is a lot of work to be done in investigating this subject, but again, homoeopathy studies the whole patient and finds that alleviation can be given with many remedies. *Salicylic acid* had been known for a long time to the homoeopaths in the treatment of tinnitus before it was used in treating rheumatic complaints in high doses. In many instances it has been found that tinnitus is one of the early side-effects of some rheumatic complaints.

Menière's disease can be helped by operation but deafness follows and as a result patients enquire if homoeopathy will relieve them. If seen early they can definitely be helped with no resultant deafness.

Another interesting point is that singers who are frequently greatly helped by throat surgeons with sprays and simple remedies for their voices or to clear up slight hoarseness, also turn to the homoeopathic physician when they realize how rapidly the right remedy works in both the acute and more chronic problems.

A minister who had to preach to a large congregation at a Special Service in Glasgow had lost his voice from acute laryngitis and did not know what to do. He then decided to call on a homoeopathic doctor there and was given *Arum triphyllum* and was amazed to find his voice so much better two hours later that he was able to speak with perfect ease and had no further trouble.

Eyes are another special branch where homoeopathy has always been able to help. Dr Compton-Burnett treated cataract, as did many of the early homoeopathic doctors, at a time when anaesthetics were not very safe and patients were unwilling to undergo surgery. Even now patients have a long time to wait before the surgeon is willing to operate and during the waiting time *Cineraria* eye drops can definitely help. In an older person vision can be maintained at an adequate level but if not, operation can now safely restore sight. Cysts round the eyelids which can be such a constantly recurring trouble are cured so often by such remedies as *Baryta carbonica*.

The tired eye and generally failing vision are undoubtedly relieved by *Ruta*. Again an acute conjunctivitis with haemorrhage is enormously benefited by *Hamamelis*. Even the retinal haemorrhages can be absorbed more quickly under this remedy and the appropriate ophthalmic surgeon's guidance.

The use of homoeopathy for eye complaints has revived and conditions which respond poorly to the modern chemico-therapeutic drugs are being greatly helped by homoeopathy. Blepharitis is often made worse by certain creams that patients use but when these are left off and patients are given such remedies as *Euphrasia* (eyebright), which has had a reputation for hundreds of years as an eye remedy, they improve; or at a worse stage will be helped so much by *Kali iodatum* (Potassium iodide).

In a threatened glaucoma one can use in addition to *Pilocarpine* drops certain remedies such as *Ledum* as well as the constitutional remedy of the patient as always.

Squints can frequently be helped by such things as *Gelsemium*, and the child may avoid operation. Again, with an obstructed tear duct in the infant, *Thiosinaminum* can clear this at once.

10

Homoeopathy on
the Farm

A homoeopathic doctor was asked by a
country veterinary surgeon if he could suggest
any remedy for a herd of Jersey cows. They were suffering
from very severe 'husk', a disease where there are small
worms present in the bronchial tubes causing a very tiresome, persistent and tearing cough, from which one or two
had already died. They were given homoeopathic *Antimonium tartaricum* mixed with their food or put into their
water and within a matter of days the herd had improved
beyond all description. Here the local vet was very much
interested and kept a bottle of this remedy to use if he met
it again. At another time the same herd developed summer
mastitis and were helped at once with *Phytolacca*. Calves
with 'husk' will also respond very well to *Antimonium
tartaricum*.

There was a well-known stable in Wiltshire whose
horses had taken many prizes in shows all over the country,
where a sudden severe outbreak of strangles took place.
This is caused by the streptococcus equinus and causes
swelling of the glands in the neck which may go on to form

abscesses. As this was increasing a homoeopathic doctor who was in the vicinity was met by the local vet to see if he could help. The doctor did not know much about horses but considering their symptoms from a homoeopathic angle he recommended *Silica* and again the vet was only too thankful to try anything as he had given heavy courses of antibiotics with no real improvement. The swelling discharged and went down within a few days and two of the horses were able to take part in a show a fortnight later.

Dogs with eczema round, or even in, the ears respond very well to *Sulphur* in a 12th or 30th potency for two or three weeks. *Arsenicum* if the hair falls off can soon stop it and *Rhus. toxicodendron* is useful when hard scabs form which do not easily fall off.

Homoeopathy is also very useful in the prevention or cure of coughs in animals, particularly in horses. It can be given to a horse to clear up his cough, but also as a preventive when horses are beginning to cough, and such remedies as *Phosphorus* will prevent others from catching it. This can be given as specially made-up powders or as tablets put into water or added to the bran mash. *Hepar sulph* is another very useful remedy for a horse who coughs after exertion as the result of dust in the hay.

Many people who keep horses also find that *Arnica* is a great help. It can be used for a horse who has had a period of strenuous racing or hunting or working and is found to be rather droopy and exhausted afterwards. A few doses of *Arnica* and he will pick up very quickly. Again this wonderful remedy is needed for bumps and bruises, for strain or even heart strain and as a rule horses need nothing further.

Nux vomica for a horse starting colic will usually stop it at once.

Rhus toxicodendron can be extremely useful for tendon strain. Horses are also apt to get bumps on their sinews from strain or a teno-synovitis and may need such remedies as *Ruta*, *Calcarea phosph* or *Hecla lava*. *Calcarea phosphorica* is a constantly needed remedy for young horses who get their legs over-strained during training and who are weakened by it.

In the 1961 epidemic of foot and mouth disease the *Daily Telegraph* above letters dealing with this disease asked —'Is the slaughter really necessary?' One of the correspondents was Mr D. W. Everitt M.P.S. then head of Nelsons Homoeopathic Pharmacy who wrote 'I am surprised that nobody, it seems, has suggested investigation by the homoeopathic method of oral vaccination against foot and mouth disease which is a virus infection—if asked I will provide *gratis* full laboratory and pharmaceutical co-operation.' In a later issue Miss Raymonde-Hawkins, Hon. Organizer Raystede Rescue Centre for Animals, Ringmer, Sussex, wrote 'Mr D. W. Everitt's suggestion is practical under British regulations. If a homoeopathic prophylactic should fail the farmer and the taxpayer will be no worse off. If it succeeds the gain would obviously be tremendous.'

In the same way that many industrial concerns tested the homoeopathic influenza oral vaccines in 1957, could we not call for, say, twelve farmers to use a homoeopathic foot and mouth vaccine. In 1961, 42,000 animals were slaughtered and the *Daily Telegraph* wrote in an editorial of this 'tragic wastefulness' and said 'the search for a prophylactic which could render cattle immune is a matter of prime importance'. The benefits of *Borax*, a likely homoeopathic remedy, were discussed. Foot and mouth disease spreads with great rapidity; and the infection can be carried by starlings and in imported meat often used in pig swill. If farmers do not boil the pig swill as suggested, a tin of contaminated meat can cause damage running into millions of pounds. The disease is endemic on the continent. Animals do not actually die of this disease, as a rule, but

live on in a condition of very ill-health, with ulcers about
the tongue, mouth, nostrils and feet. Now, all these
symptoms are covered in *Borax*, an old domestic remedy
which has had full homoeopathic proving. Might not it be
possible for someone in authority to give *Borax* pro-
phylactically in a district known to have foot and mouth
disease. In Dr Margaret Tyler's *Homoeopathic Drug Picture*
we have under *Borax* 'Aphthae on mouth and on tongue
and on inner surface of cheek, bleeding easily with great
heat and dryness of mouth with cracked tongue. Phagedenic
ulcers on joints of fingers and toes'. *Borax* is one of the
sodium salts whose symptoms are worse in cold, and the
outbreak in 1961 started during the cold wet weather of
October and in 1967 the same. Cows have another *Borax*
symptom in that they do not like going down a ramp if at
all steep—a fear of downward movement is a strong
indication for using the drug.

Borax is absolutely safe to use in drinking water for
animals and it is very easy to administer. It is an interesting
fact that although such drastic measures are used to wipe
out an epidemic of foot and mouth, *The Times* in December
1960 said 'the foot and mouth situation is not clearing up
as quickly as could be expected', quoting a statement from
the Ministry of Agriculture. 'During the past week there
had been a disappointing increase in outbreaks.'

In an outbreak of foot and mouth disease in Switzerland
in 1960 Dr Pierre Schmidt of Geneva, the present 'Father
of Homoeopathy' reported that a veterinary 'pupil' of his
had 'magnificent results' with homoeopathic prophylactic
treatment in cattle. They were given two appropriate
nosodes in the 30, 200 and 1m potencies, two doses of each
potency for three days running, and after that *Nitric acid* 6c
was added to the water in the drinking trough. The use of
Nitric acid is analogous to the use of, say, *Belladonna* in the
prophylaxis of scarlet fever, for the symptoms induced by

this drug in provings bear a close similarity to those of foot and mouth disease.

It is important to note that none of the animals treated in this way developed the disease although they were dosed and looked after by the same cowman who cared for the infected herd.

Dr Schmidt has suggested that it would be wise to make fresh nosode potencies each year because of possible variation in the strain of 'germs epidemicus'. As he says, saliva from infected animals in regions where the disease is still rife could be used. This might be a practical possibility in Europe where the disease is so prevalent and the Homoeopathic International League could sponsor such an enquiry.

There is a long history of the use of homoeopathy for treating animals.

An interesting account is given by a farmer in Ireland of his experience with homoeopathy in animals. When he first inherited his estate he was very pleased to find a book of his great-grandfather's and a box of homoeopathic tinctures all carefully preserved with instructions about what they were for and how to use them for the different animals. There is a list of remedies which were given in 1951.

> For fits in foxhound puppies—*Tarentula*. As a prophylactic against distemper in foxhound puppies *Gelsemium* 3X (winter jasmine). These were given in tablets twice a week.
> For Bovine tuberculosis—*Drosera* 30 (made from sundew) last thing at night every 3rd day.
> For Fowl Paralysis—*Argentum nitricum* 6X.
> For chronic mastitis in cows—*Eupatorium perfoliatum* 30.

An account was also given of a famous hunter who at the age of twelve years became suddenly so lame that the vet suggested having him put down. However the owner, who loved this horse, immediately rang his friend who prescribed homoeopathic remedies, and he sent *Rhus toxicodendron* for the animal. Within a week he was very much better and had lost his lameness. He hunted as well as ever and every Christmas a card arrived 'with love from Midnight, still going strong'. At the age of nineteen this horse had another bout of lameness which was once more cured in two or three weeks by *Rhus toxicodendron* and he went on at full work until he was twenty-two.

Rheumatism is a complaint met with in horses and usually responds to one of four remedies—*Bryonia*, *Rhus. toxicodendron*, *Aconite* and *Nux vomica*.

There was the case of a horse aged sixteen, with rather bad rheumatism in his back which made it difficult for him to work. In the history there was uncertainty as to whether he was better or worse for movement and *Rhus toxicodendron* was tried as the first remedy. At the end of a fortnight he was not any better. Reporting on the horse it was remarked by the vet, that special note had been made as to whether or not he was better for movement. It had been definitely established that he was perfectly all right after having two days rest. On the strength of this report he was sent *Bryonia* 30 and did very well, and we find that a 30th potency is generally the most efficient for any animal when prescribed for over a period of time.

Inflammation may occur from wounds and strains and the use of *Aconite*, when there is fever, greatly hastens healing.

Influenza in horses is most prevalent in the spring and autumn and is generally ushered in by symptoms like those of catarrh with general fever—a watery discharge from the nose which soon becomes thick and sometimes has blood in it; the eyes may be inflamed and the glands of the jaw and throat are often enlarged so that swallowing is difficult and obviously painful. This is often accompanied by a degree of weakness. An initial treatment of *Aconite* may quickly clear it up. *Mercurius vivus* will be needed if a sore throat is accompanied by sweating, watery eyes and intolerance to light. *Belladonna* is especially indicated when the eyes are inflamed and there is inability to swallow even fluids. *Arsenicum* can be called for if there is great weakness and loose and probably blood streaked evacuations, and *Bryonia* is needed when *Aconite* has not stopped the fever and breathing is becoming difficult.

In acute indigestion in animals homoeopathy can give very rapid results. If cattle begin to eat green fodder when they are not used to it, a condition called Hoven or 'Blown' can result. It is common for cattle to eat a quantity which is far more than the stomach can cope with. A great deal of gas is generated, sometimes so rapidly that the animal may die before relief can be given. If it persists an opening may have to be made in the stomach, but if it is discovered in time *Colchicum autumnale* (autumn crocus) can give relief in a very short time and is often sufficient to produce a cure without having to make an opening to let out the wind. Some animals get great distension from a sensitivity to green food, even in small quantities, and this may occur during the season when scarcely anything but green food is given. In these cases *Arsenicum* or *Nux vomica* hardly ever fails to produce a cure. In less acute cases colic is produced by unsuitable food; exposure to cold and wet will also bring it on. Colic is said to occur more rarely in cows than in horses and it is found that for either *Aconite* gives rapid relief. *Arsenicum* may also be needed to follow, particularly if the attack has been produced by green food or cold water after sweating. The third remedy that may be called for here is *Nux vomica* which is so frequently found to be a useful animal medicine.

An incident was sent recently by a patient which the writer

thought might interest those who were investigating homoeopathy. In 1951 her sister-in-law had two turkey oaks with oozing wounds sucked by flies and moths. When in leaf they were watered by homoeopathic *Manganese* in low potency. In 1952 one tree appeared to be cured and the other had only a slight oozing wound. In August 1952 *Manganese* 6 was given and later *Sulphur* 6 to both trees by watering round their roots. In 1953 there was a slight oozing again and No. 1 tree was watered with *Mercurius* 6 and No. 2 with *Mercurius* 30. Both were quickly much better but No. 2 was not quite so good as No. 1. No. 2 was then given *Mercurius* 6. In November the owner of the trees wrote 'they are very well and no sign of that oozing at all. No. 2 tree had an enormous crop of acorns and the other not so many, and since they had none last year it looks as if this has done a "cure" '. From that time they have flourished.

The same family are very keen on treating gardens and trees in poor condition with homoeopathic trace elements. Recently they had a field where the ground was in such a poor condition, due to neglect by the former owner, that everyone said they would never grow a crop of anything on it. So the couple went out with a homoeopathic mixture of *Boron* in water in a very low potency and although the neighbours thought they were mad they watered part of the field with it. The result was a bumper crop of wheat. Their one regret after was that they had done only half the field and left the other half as it was so as to prove the effects of their 'treatment'. With proper crop rotation the productivity of the field should return to normal.

I I

Homoeopathic
Teaching

For many years, the Homoeopathic Faculty in London has been the world centre for teaching homoeopathy. Every year the Honeyman-Gillespie and the Compton-Burnett lectures are given by leading homoeopaths between September of one year and June of the following year. In addition to these lectures, there are out-patients' clinics, ward rounds to attend, and a great deal of individual teaching in the adjoining Hospital. Many of those who attend have become Associates of the Faculty of Homoeopathy, or have taken the examination and become Members of the Faculty.

It is also most interesting to notice the number of doctors who come from all over the world. We have had doctors from Bermuda, one from Chile, and we have in fact, had wonderful contacts with several doctors in South America as well as several from San Francisco, from Vancouver and other parts of Canada. In recent years doctors have attended from Italy, Switzerland, Norway, Denmark and Holland, and at the International Homoeopathic League meetings the French and German homoeopaths take a great part.

In the early days of my experience many students came from India and spent a year attending lectures and clinics. I always enjoyed teaching them either on my ward rounds or in the out-patients' department and clinics and with the weekly lecture. They came from varying backgrounds and had an extraordinary knowledge of actual homoeopathic remedies and gained a lot of clinical experience during their time in Britain. Many have become Associates or Members of the Faculty of Homoeopathy. A number of them took the diploma examination of the Faculty as they were not eligible for membership. This increased their standing on returning to their own country. Again, many of these have improved the standard of homoeopathy and its practice in India to such an extent that the Indian Government has now recognized this form of medicine and given Homoeopathic Medical Schools recognition and financial help. We do not see so many of our Indian colleagues at the long courses nowadays, although many who are in practice in London attend the short courses.

In the last few years a number of doctors have come from Australia to learn homoeopathy and many have gone back, some British doctors joining them, so that today in Sydney, Melbourne and Queensland there is increasing interest. This carries on a long standing tradition of homoeopathic medicine in the Antipodes. There used to be a family of homoeopathic doctors in Sydney by the name of Dick, and one of my most faithful patients met homoeopathy through their treatment, and has been enthusing about it ever since. It is frequently found now that some of our keenest support comes from homoeopathic doctors in Australia who have attended courses in this country, and some have decided to remain and practise here. There have also been doctors from New Zealand, and increasing interest in Canada. They have been finding a useful dialogue with their colleagues in the United States of America. Although often very isolated, the doctors in Canada maintain their interest and find their homoeopathic results very rewarding.

We have had over the last few years a steady stream of doctors from America. This is very encouraging, for at one time, America was the leading country in teaching homoeopathic methods, and our doctors went there to study with Dr Kent in Chicago. There were also various homoeopathic hospitals in the USA, which have gradually been taken over by orthodox medicine even though retaining their title of homoeopathic. The American doctors seem very impressed with our intensive courses, and the climate of medicine in the USA is becoming once again more understanding towards homoeopathic principles, so that the American Institute of Homoeopathy is growing fast and adding to its numbers all the time.

This strong lay and medical support makes it more difficult for the United States Food and Drug Administration to refuse to recognize homoeopathic medicines.

There is now a Mexican Homoeopathic School where they teach a basic medical curriculum and introduce homoeopathic therapeutics to the senior students. In South America generally, there is a great deal of teaching being done by some leading homoeopaths. The wide acceptance of this form of medicine in Argentina inspires some of the doctors to come to London for post-graduate instruction. Doctors have also come from Chile, although practice there is much more isolated. In the Far East we have a Centre for Homoeopathy in Tokyo. And it is widely practised in the USSR.

There are either members or corresponding members all over Europe. Paris of course, has always been a stronghold since Hahnemann spent the last years of his life and died there.

After Hahnemann's death, each country developed its own application of homoeopathy, and without Hahnemann's lasting and directing influence, it was bound to lose some of its original dependence on the basic Principle that he advocated. In Germany homoeopathy has always flourished, although the national characteristic has influenced its development.

The oldest and probably most revered practitioner of homoeopathy today is Dr Pierre Schmidt of Geneva who adheres very closely to the original principles enunciated and taught by Hahnemann. In 1925 he and Dr Thuinzing of Holland had the excellent idea of forming an International Homoeopathic League. This League continues to meet every year or two in order to exchange ideas and experiences in homoeopathy. The first meeting actually took place in Holland, where there has always been a small, but strong nucleus of homoeopathic doctors. This has served to help those more isolated, in that they all join the League as individual members, irrespective of the strength of their national group. The fiftieth anniversary of the League was held in Rotterdam in April 1975. The importance of the International League is increasing closer liaison in Europe since the formation of the Common Market. This is of particular importance with professional groups because of the recognition of the standard of education across national boundaries.

The more immediate problem to us as homoeopaths is the acceptance and recognition of the homoeopathically prepared remedies. Hahnemann himself, who was an expert chemist, laid down rules for the collection and preparation of the substances that he investigated. These rules were closely followed by those in the United States chiefly, who, at the time, confirmed his findings and extended the *Materia Medica*. The pharmacists of the International League are playing an ever important role in establishing the basic methods of preparation of the mother tinctures which must be adhered to for a substance to be included in the International Homoeopathic Pharmacopoeia. Both America and Britain have their own homoeopathic pharmacopoeias which are generally recognized in their own countries (the USA pharmacopoeia was established in 1925). This is generally true of France and Germany, although each country has slightly different criteria of extraction, preparation and potentization. When homoeopathy was in its infancy, many doctors prepared their own remedies, but nowadays with increased specialization, they rely on the pharmacists to provide reliable preparations, so it is essential that an agreed basic principle in the making of the remedies should be established internationally. The freedom of the doctor to choose the potency with which he can do most good must be safe-guarded. Britain is playing a leading role in all these discussions both within the homoeopathic pharmaceutical industry, and amongst pharmacists generally and many more pharmacists are becoming pharmaceutical associates of the Faculty of Homoeopathy in Great Britain.

The International League provides a meeting place for pharmacists and doctors and has recently attracted a great deal more interest among dentists and veterinary surgeons and other paramedical personnel—so the scientific interest is growing. The League provides a 'Club' where research can be discussed in detail. This role of the League will almost certainly be more important in the future.

One of the early students attending a long course— that is, a year's teaching—was a woman doctor from Athens. She absorbed the teaching avidly and did a magnificent exam for the Membership of the Faculty of Homoeopathy. When she went back, she managed to interest a number of doctors in Greece, so that, in turn, she became their leader and influenced the medical students of the local university. As a result a small School of Homoeopathy has been started. Great impetus was given to this by the International League Meeting in Athens which was honoured by the presence of state dignitaries. Since then, interest among the undergraduates has continued to increase, and a useful exchange of information is being maintained through the post-graduate School of Homoeopathy.

For many years Brussels has been a centre of homoeopathy led to Dr Schepens. His son has continued in the tradition and has taken his examination for membership of the Faculty in this country.

Vienna is another very active centre for European homoeopathy. Correspondence is being carried on between orthodox practices and the ever increasing number of homoeopathic doctors, and opportunities for study are offered there to any doctors who may be interested.

We find in London too, that we get a representative group of doctors coming each year to our Courses of Instruction. In recent years doctors and students from over twenty countries have attended the courses.

However, when Dr Quin first introduced homoeopathy to England, there was very little teaching of the standardization of medicine. Much medical discussion took place in open debate and the lay public were often present. Homoeopathy was debated at such meetings and the lay audience took hold of this form of therapy, there being very little else at the time. They learnt the *Materia Medica* and wrote pamphlets on its use in practice. Dr Quin countered this as he thought it was usurping the right of the physician. Medicine was learned at that time by attaching oneself to an eminent physician as an apprentice, and homoeopathy spread by this means. However when Dr Quin formed the Homoeopathic Society to safeguard the professionalism of homoeopathic medicine, he was also the instigator of the opening of the formal School of Homoeopathic Medicine in association with the

Hospital. It was a deliberate proposal that this should be post-graduate so that the basic medical training would be undertaken at a recognized university under university teachers. For thirty-five years Quin was both the leading light in the Society and in the teaching of homoeopathy. A Hahnemannian lecture always opened each session and some of the great teachers were Dr Dudgeon, Dr Richard Hughes, and later Dr Clarke, and of course Dr Compton-Burnett. The School of Homoeopathy was always a centre for debate but the emphasis was on principles and the basic *Materia Medica*. There were formal monthly meetings of the Society at which lectures were given and published in a quarterly journal.

Besides this there were series of informal lectures given to interested students on homoeopathic *Materia Medica*. Later the organization became more academic when Dr Margaret Tyler became Dean. She ran a very successful correspondence course which was sent to many parts of the world. She also used to love to have students and young doctors in her out-patients' clinics and taught them a great deal. In the last century her father built a wing to the London Homoeopathic Hospital and created a number of teaching scholarships which enabled British doctors to go to study with Dr Kent in Chicago. They came back very stimulated and were able to undertake more intensive lectures and teaching in Britain.

There was a period between 1930 and 1950 when students of homoeopathy were fewer because of the vast improvement in public health and hygiene and the introduction of some of the modern chemical drugs. Yet, when Dr C. E. Wheeler's *Principles and Practice of Homoeopathy* was written and published in 1940, it was seized upon by those interested and widely read. At that time, the *Homoeopathic Journal* was published regularly and was full of practical advice and recorded the useful discussions following the monthly meetings of the Society. Dr Tyler brought out a journal called *Homoeopathy* and she also collected lectures and articles of interest from all over the world.

A series of very good teaching lectures was given each year at the Hospital. Dr Borland gave the Honeyman-Gillespie series each year, and these were invaluable. Sir John Weir gave the Compton-Burnett lectures on the Principles and Practice of Homoeopathy, Dr C. E. Wheeler gave weekly lectures on Remedies, their origin and early history and provings and there were other lectures, and speakers.

It is an interesting fact that whole families would support and sponsor this type of medical teaching. Through the years, there have been many patrons who have helped and continue to support the homoeopathic cause.

The number of homoeopathic physicians in this country remained about the same in spite of modern advances in therapy, so the interest was maintained. With the passing of the Faculty of Homoeopathy Act in 1950 it then became necessary to reassess the teaching responsibilities invested in the Faculty and Hospital. The development of post graduate education amongst physicians generally has become increasingly necessary as medicine has become more and more complicated. Since Dr Quin first insisted that homoeopathy be practised only by registered medical practitioners in order to maintain recognition of the Faculty on these grounds, it was necessary to tighten up the rules for students. Previously, students were accepted who were recognized as eligible to practice medicine in their own countries. This gave the British School of Homoeopathy an international standing of which it is very proud. However, the membership of the Faculty of Homoeopathy is now open only to doctors eligible to practise medicine in Great Britain.

The training of the General Practitioner in homoeo-

pathic therapeutics has become particularly important
over the last ten years. It has always been the medicine of
the whole person, whereas the tendency in modern
medicine has been to narrow down the field of the doctors'
interest. With the ever increasing specialization, the patient
seems to have been forgotten. In this country, the General
Practitioner, having felt rather unimportant within this
scientific revolution of mechanistic medicine, has gradually
come into his own, as the doctor who cares for the whole
patient in his environment. This is largely due to a group
of doctors who have pioneered the College of General
Practitioners which has been recognized since 1970 by
becoming The Royal College of General Practitioners.

A doctor can regain this concept of the patient as needing
medical help by studying homoeopathic medicine which
treats the patient together with his pathology.

Since the early 1960's, there have been Intensive Courses
of Homoeopathic Medicine lasting a week, three times a
year. These have included introductory lectures for the new
doctor and have incorporated the *Materia Medica* lectures
and lectures on the Principles and Practice of Homoeopathy
which has always been part of the teaching of this school of
medicine. One thing that has been invaluable has been
the exchange of their experiences in homoeopathic practice
among the new doctors who attend. This body of experience
of the action of homoeopathy has added up-to-date clinical
material establishing the efficiency of homoeopathic
medicine in the 20th century.

The training of doctors in homoeopathy has always
been individual and some can spare a longer time than
others for its study. Lectures and teaching continue throughout the year based at the Royal London Homoeopathic
Hospital, and training is also given in teaching homoeopathic practices. The patients are very cooperative and often
take a real interest and participate in the learning process,

appreciating the fact that the doctors present are learning homoeopathy. There is not the usual feeling of being just 'an object' but of really taking an active part in increasing their chances of getting well. This does not apply to a *Natrum mur.* who may easily resent the questions or having to talk in company! However, this in itself gives a wonderful guide to the prescribers, as would a *Pulsatilla* patient who loves company, fuss, and opportunity for full outpourings of troubles to an attentive audience!

These courses are obviously appreciated by the doctors who are coming in ever increasing numbers. The doctors' interests are aroused by their colleagues who urge them to attend courses from all over the country, but what is more striking now, is that the patients themselves are asking doctors for homoeopathic treatment, and when asked how they can learn, they are told about the courses in London.

Weekend courses are also held in Glasgow three times a year and more doctors are attending each time.

Regional meetings are also arranged in various parts of the country and there is a British Homoeopathic Congress held every two years where established homoeopathic practitioners discuss problems of mutual interest relevant to the medicine of their day.

None of this teaching of homoeopathy would be available without the valuable help and support of the Homoeopathic Research and Educational Trust. This was initiated at the time of the Faculty of Homoeopathy Act when the charitable funds originally administered by the Homoeopathic Society were transferred to this Trust. The Trust also encourages and supports individual research projects and general teaching.

In 1975, for the first time, medical students from all the teaching hospitals were invited to London. It is hoped to extend this throughout the country. The interest shown establishes the need for a safe alternative method of treatment.

12

Twentieth Century Homoeopaths

I have known many of the renowned homoeopaths of the twentieth century, and would like to give a short account of some of them.

The first I would like to mention was Dr James Compton-Burnett, who was my uncle, but who died before my time. He had studied medicine in Vienna but came back to Britain to take his Glasgow MB in 1872. He was another who became very dissatisfied with the medical practice of his day and thought of giving up in order to do something more useful. Fortunately, he was persuaded to look into homoeopathy before refuting it, and was so impressed by a book on the subject by Dr Richard Hughes, that he began to apply its principles straight away. Because of his inclination and training in clinical analyses he found the logic and testing of homoeopathic concepts a practical means of benefiting mankind. As a physician he realized that a new field was opened to him; a field so vast that it included all the ailments, and their cures, to which man is subject. He published a number of striking monographs, one of which on *Natrum muriaticum* is very popular with the doctors new to homoeopathy. Two other useful ones were *Diseases of the Spleen with Ceanothus* and *Diseases of the Liver with Chelidonium.* These show that drugs which are poisonous to certain organs can be used in small doses to stimulate those same organs. Dr Compton-Burnett also worked with great enthusiasm and interest on the long proved disease products for the treatment and cure of disease. Hahnemann had already introduced *Psorinum*, a preparation made from scabies, *Medorrhinum* from gonorrhoea and *Lueticum* from syphilis, in addition to these preparations *Lyssin* was prepared from the saliva of a mad dog before Pasteur did in France and Dr Swann also developed *Anthracinum* from anthrax. As early as 1871, Dr Swann prepared his *Tuberculinum* from tuberculosis sputum, while Dr Compton-Burnett had a special preparation from TB sputum which he called *Bacillinum*. Both these preparations in connection with TB had been used for many years before Koch and his work were ever heard of.

In 1886, Dr Compton-Burnett wrote 'There are but few viruses known to science that I have not used as therapeutic agents'. Thus it will be seen that homoeopathy was far ahead of other branches of medicine in using disease products for the cure of disease.

Then there was Dr Skinner, one of the leading homoeopathic doctors at the end of the 19th century. I never knew him but I looked after various relations of his for the last years of their lives. One of his sisters, when she died, left me his cases of homoeopathic medicines which I have found invaluable. He was born and educated in Edinburgh and destined for a commercial career. But this didn't at all suit him and he started on the study of medicine in 1849. In 1857 he became MD of the University of St Andrews where he had already obtained the gold medal of Sir James Simpson's class. Dr Skinner's pre-eminence in the speciality of diseases of women and obstetrics singled him out for Simpson's notice and he was taken into his practice as his private assistant for two years. Sir James was always the first of Dr Skinner's medical heroes and his regard for him increased with time. Before Dr Skinner accepted the assistant-ship he asked the advice of a friend who knew Sir James very well. 'Simpson' said the friend, 'has a heart as big as a pumpkin and the temper of the very devil'. Skinner decided that for the sake of the big heart he would risk the temper and accepted the post.

About two and a half years before Skinner started his medical studies Simpson had read his first paper on chloroform anaesthesia before the Medico-Chirurgical Society of Edinburgh. This met with a storm of opposition, but was soon overcome and in Skinner's day Simpson's triumph was complete. Skinner always retained his enthusiasm for chloroform anaesthesia and invented the convenient inhaler (Skinner's mask) and drop bottle (Skinner's drop-bottle).

Skinner's relationship with Simpson is important from the homoeopathic aspect as he learned from Sir James the value of giving only one remedy at a time and it speaks highly for Skinner's character, that he maintained such intimate relations with one who was undoubtedly among the leading medical lights of his century. Dr Skinner went on to Liverpool where he enjoyed a busy consulting practice for a number of years. Then his health broke down and he was practically *hors de combat* for three years with intractable sleeplessness, constipation and severe acidity of the stomach and he felt unable to do any work.

He then became acquainted with Dr Berridge, a homoeopathic physician to whom he expressed an interest in homoeopathy. The up-shot of this was that Dr Berridge prescribed *Sulphur* in the highest possible potency and its effect was a revelation to Dr Skinner. He said 'I shall never forget the marvellous change which the first dose effected in a few weeks, especially the rolling-away, as it were, of a dense and heavy cloud from my mind'. He was cured of his constipation and acid dyspepsia, sleeplessness, deficient assimilation and debility and restored to a life of usefulness and vigour.

He then took up the study of homoeopathy in earnest using as his text-books *The Organan*, *Materia Medica Pura*, and *Chronic Diseases* of Hahnemann. He was advised by Dr Berridge to get two or three dozen remedies in the 30th potency and give them only when he was sure he had found the *similimum*. These he used rather secretly until he was sure of his ground. He then publicly announced his changed practice and resigned from membership of the Liverpool Medical Institute. He had practised for twenty years as an allopath but in 1875 found himself compelled to start work afresh. He adopted homoeopathy whole-heartedly and the homoeopaths of his day gladly gave him their support. He said that he took up the keystone of the triumphal arch *similia similibus curentur* and the piers and buttresses of the arch: first, one single medicine at a time, and second, that only in an infinitesimal dose. Every man must decide for himself according to the light that is in him and be guided by experience as to what is the infinitesimal dose. But as Professor Frost in the *Hahnemannian Monthly* of 1873 puts it 'if the right remedy be given in large or in smaller or even in infinitesimal doses a cure will result in many cases'.

At the end of last century Skinner became a member of the Dining Club which consisted of Dr Compton-Burnett, Dr Robert Cooper, Dr Skinner and Dr Clarke. This was organized by Dr Cooper and was later known as the Cooper Club. Dr Cooper was an ardent homoeopath whose enormous knowledge of many unusual remedies was infinitely helpful in Dr Clarke's compilation of his dictionary. These four men approached the problem of treatment from the strictly Hahnemannian standpoint; indications first and the name of the disease second.

Dr Cooper's son Dr Le Hunte Cooper was a keen homoeopath like his father and did a lot of original work on the possible poisonous effects of cooking in aluminium and the effects of homoeopathic *Alumina* in treatment.

Having had the privilege of knowing some of the giants of homoeopathy in the last thirty or forty years, the first person I got to know well was Dr John Henry Clarke who succeeded Dr Compton-Burnett as editor of *Homoeopathic World*.

He graduated from Edinburgh and was appointed physician to the London Homoeopathic Hospital and lecturer to the Homoeopathic School of that time. His whole approach to homoeopathy was in its clinical aspect. The homoeopathic *Materia Medica* at the turn of the century was imperfect, although it dealt with the symptoms of proved drugs, but provings of the newer drugs were very scattered and not easily obtainable.

Clarke spent sixteen years of monumental work in collecting all available knowledge of drugs into one *Dictionary of Materia Medica*. The dictionary was devised to present the picture of each remedy so that it could be recognized. He used clinical symptoms and felt that objections to them were academic rather than practical and it is an invaluable work in practice today. When I was very young, Dr Clarke used to invite me to accompany him to the Royal Society of Medicine. I always remember the first occasion, when a fellow hospital house physician, afterwards my partner, lent me a necklace and insisted on my wearing my most elegant dress; and how she and another houseman saw me off from the hospital doorstep in a style they considered fitting for such an occasion. I went to the Royal Society several times with Dr Clarke, and he sent me two families of patients whom I have looked after until now.

Clarke revelled in controversy, and for years took the opposite views to Dr Richard Hughes. Then Dr Charles Wheeler became a new pleader for homoeopathy. He was a very charming man and an excellent speaker and it was a wonderful experience to work with him. He liked to start his ward rounds at 8.30, and always arrived half an hour earlier to have breakfast with his House Physician. It was well worth while being ready at this early hour, as his talk was not only very interesting, but also very instructive. He had an inexhaustible knowledge of drugs, where they came from, who had discovered them, and other bits of information. He had a great influence upon homoeopaths for many years and he augmented the pathological arguments of Richard Hughes with the more subtle appeal of biology.

Wheeler revived Hahnemann's concept of vital reaction to disease and drugs, and restated it in terms of modern biology. He wrote in an address to the Homoeopathic Association on *A Hundred Years of Homoeopathy*:

'Homoeopathy is not a theory, involves no dogmatic faith. It is a simple rule of practice applied to a particular sphere of medicine. The treatment of the sick by drugs. There have been endless attempts to explain why the rule should work, and many speculations from Hahnemann onwards, but the one cry of the homoeopath from Hahnemann's day has been "You do not need, you are not asked, to believe this explanation because I say so, or in deference to any theoretical explanation of life processes such as was proved for instance behind the Galenical practices—I assert that this rule works only because I have tried it over and over again". He said later that "our heresy" is not a theory but a rule of practice which is surviving, and increasing today. He showed by experimentation that drugs can stimulate the defensive mechanisms of the body, even to the production of agglutinins in the case of *Baptisia*, and demonstrated the action of *Phosphorus*, *Veratrum viride* and others on the opsonic index. He pointed out the relation of the enhanced activity of the homoeopathic potencies to the colloidal state, emphasizing the fact that certain agents in a great state of subdivision stimulate fervent action, which in stronger solutions inhibit, thus bearing out the Arndt-Schultz law.

Dr Wheeler also said that 'his belief in infinitesimals was not a fad but the result of rigorous experiment—even more rigorous than that applied to most new claims just because those claims are so difficult to accept. What we believe we believe on experimental grounds, what so many disbelieve, they disbelieve on no grounds but those of a prior unlikelihood and a refusal to put their prejudice to the test'. In every development there is no doubt that however fantastic, Hahnemann worked not by theory, but by experiment and observation.

As the early followers of Hahnemann used to advise: —'Don't think—*try*.' Homoeopathic potentization was also explained very clearly in Dr Wheeler's introduction to his *Principles and Practice of Homoeopathy*. The remedies he saw, according to the principles of homoeopathy are prepared quite simply, but the greatest care has to be taken so that the best prepared tinctures and potencies can be produced.

The name of Sir John Weir need hardly be enlarged upon, as he is already so well known in the field of homoeopathy. However, as I knew him personally over many years, I should like to pay tribute to him. He was a great homoeopathic teacher and prescriber and was ever anxious to help anyone who needed it. He gave the Compton-Burnett lectures each year and the great interest of his life was homoeopathy. When he celebrated his fiftieth anniversary as a physician to the Royal London Homoeopathic Hospital, a banquet was held at the Savoy, and their Royal Highnesses the Duke and Duchess of Gloucester honoured the evening with their presence. Dr Stuart

McAusland from Liverpool, and Dr Douglas Ross from Glasgow, on behalf of their Liverpool and Scottish colleagues, honoured and praised Sir John's teaching—his patience, his sympathy in dealing with his patients, and the doctors studying homoeopathy. Dr Ross told of his personal triumph in visiting America. Dr Ross said of him 'no one has a better grasp of essentials and a quicker eye for detail—and all controlled by his strong Scottish common sense'. Dr Frank Bodman of Bristol, who is our leading homoeopathic doctor in the southwest of England, also paid tribute. Sir John, he said, had expressed the fact that he did not like anything flattering said to his face, as it was painful for him to be praised, but on that occasion we all had to tell him how much we admired him!

Dr Borland was another homoeopathic doctor to whom I was house physician, and later assistant in the out-patient department. He was a superb teacher—especially over a cup of coffee following his ward rounds! He had been in Salonika and then Upper Armenia in the 1914–18 War as a very young man and his health was permanently weakened by his experiences in charge of a Field Hospital. He was in charge of the Royal London Homoeopathic Hospital in the 1939–45 War and one time was blown out of bed by a bomb which hit the nearby Nurses' Home.

On his ward rounds, Dr Borland would stop beside the bed of a very ill child or some other patient and not speak for a minute or two. Then after examining the patient, he would first ask me what I wanted to give, and then he would tell me what he was sure the patient needed. I can recall his pausing at the door again and again, to say 'Go back and look at that patient several times today. Get him into your head, he is the perfect picture of such and such a drug'. He never minded being rung up for advice and he gave a series of Honeyman-Gillespie lectures on homoeopathy of which I still have the notes. I find them invaluable.

He wrote several small books on pneumonia and digestive remedies, children's types, and others which are again, still extremely useful today at courses in our homoeopathic teaching.

Dr Borland was one of the four physicians who, with Sir John Weir, were given a Sir Henry Tyler Scholarship and went to America to study homoeopathy under Dr Kent in Chicago. They re-enforced the concept of the drug picture, that is, Hahnemann's 'totality of characteristic symptoms in the patient', and 'the drug which must match if cure is to result'.

Dr Borland always liked us to see patients as drugs when we had a good drug picture—the result was that when I went to a theatre with another young homoeopathic doctor, we had a wonderful time. A father arrived with three children, the youngest of whom was a boy of about ten and they sat in front of us. The father looked very irritable, and the eldest child told the boy not to worry him, but when the youngest could not resist asking questions any longer, he was well sat upon—we turned to each other and said *Nux*! A girl, two rows in front of us, was quite definitely unhappy about something, and as we watched, she managed to change places with everyone until she was sitting on the gangway, she obviously hated being closed in, and we suggested *Argentum nitricum* as her remedy. Then we prescribed for the different actors and actresses and were quite amazed at the number of counter-parts we had in practice as patients, and oh, how we enjoyed 'suggesting their drug!'

I have kept this habit ever since, and find myself unconsciously prescribing for a man walking in front of me, on his deliberate walk, his obvious meaning to arrive at his destination, to whom I should give *Natrum muriaticum*. Or the twittery, obviously nervous, but very neat, old lady who hesitates at the road crossing, whom I deduce needs *Arsenicum*, and so it goes on, but this all adds great interest to homoeopathic prescribing.

After the War Dr W. E. Boyd of Glasgow attempted to discover the nature of the stimulus with which homoeopathic drugs in potency affect the defences of the body. He physically demonstrated (to the satisfaction of the Horder Committee) that drugs in infinitesimal subdivision do exhibit some form of energy, and research is still in progress.

Dr Margaret Tyler was another wonderfully keen homoeopath. She had a great gift for writing, and her *Drug Pictures* is a very breezy book; quite individual, and still very popular. She was a very good teacher in out-patients, and for many years ran a clinic for mentally handicapped children on a Monday morning, at which I assisted her. She was particularly interested in children and worked very closely with the NSPCC and achieved some unbelievably good results. She suggested *Natrum muriaticum* for the backward and difficult child who was very late in talking and apt to sleep-walk, *Baryta carbonica* for the dull, heavy child, who was obviously slow and backward; the child who looked 'rather mental', and who often had a tendency to enlarged glands and sore throats. *Medorrhinum* for the Mongol child, *Tuberculinum bovinum* for children who were resentful, and then *Staphisagria* which can be useful for the very resentful, but easily hurt child, and *Capsicum* for the homesick.

It was her father, Sir Henry Tyler, who created scholarships to send a number of men to study homoeopathy in the U.S.A.

Dr Elizabeth Wright Hubbard of New York was a very experienced and famous homoeopath. She came for an intensive course in London in the mid-sixties and gave daily lectures to the enquiring doctors. She also gave the monthly address to the Faculty of Homoeopathy during the Course week and the meeting was packed to the doors.

She lectured on remedies with comparisons such as between *Psorinum* and *Medorrhinum*.

She gave a talk on what she called 'Pitfalls' where she urged those who were interested in homoeopathy to take the patients case properly and to put extra work into it; if necessary to use a Repertory, and read it up in one of the *Materia Medica* by Kent, Clarke or Margaret Tyler. She advised doctors on what books they should read when really learning about a remedy, and advised them particularly to note the mental and general symptoms first. Then the strange, rare, and peculiar symptoms, a pathological symptom such as warts, and the tissue and organ most affected. She urged them also to remember the pathology in the light of the sources of our remedies, whether mineral or animal. In describing the endocrine systems she would give a most telling picture of a remedy in quite a few words and I constantly remember her description of *Psorinum* with its hay-fever in spring: headaches which are better for eating: constipation in infants. She described the green acrid discharge of *Psorinum* worse for draughts, the history of never being well since, and the fourteen to twenty-one day periodicity so constantly found in patients needing this drug; full of complaints 'as if'. She described the chilly patient who always wraps up and wears a woollen scarf round his head; the babies who play all day and scream all night. 'Psorinum patients' she said 'could be described as the great unwashable', and this patient, she ended, suffers more with less cause than anyone else described in the *Materia Medica*. Dr Wright Hubbard died in 1967 and is a great loss to the homoeopathic cause.

All these men and women and the so many more who could be named have forcibly brought forth the importance of homoeopathy over the past few years.

13

The Contemporary Scene

Homoeopathy is not a philosophy, it is a principle.

Conventional medicine changes as the scientist probes deeper and deeper into what goes on in the living body. The evolution of modern pathology has come about through the invention of increasingly sophisticated laboratory equipment, yet nothing that has been learned of the subtle workings of the human body has invalidated the original Hahnemannian concepts of symptoms and analyses.

In light of the modern technical advances the original provings have been tested and re-examined in America and in Britain by homoeopathic provers, and this has continued to be the backbone of homoeopathic therapeutics all based upon observation and results.

The pharmacist is a chemical engineer who uses the laboratory to investigate a substance and its effects. Thus the explosion of the sulphonamides, the antibiotics, the tranquillizers, the diuretics, the muscle relaxants, and antispasmodics. Drug firms have long been aware of the value of indigenous medicines and have always sought the active ingredients that contributed to its effectiveness. The chemist will purify this to apply it to modern practice.

Modern medicine is very exciting and has done a great deal to alleviate suffering and pain. Amongst the greatest benefactors of symptom relief were asthmatics. Some chemical helps such as adrenalin, sodium cromoglycate and cortisone brought great comfort until the patient built up a resistance to the relief. This relief was nevertheless no greater than that found in the homoeopathic treatment of asthmatic conditions, except that at the end of the homoeo-pathic treatment the patient was generally cured.

Individual differences in response to some of the chemo-therapeutic agents used in tuberculosis treatments led physicians to discover more about enzyme pathways and the importance of genetic considerations in drug metabolism. This shows how complicated drug therapy is at the moment. Drug interactions are an important con-sideration and this is constantly being brought to the attention of the medical profession. What a drug is shown to do in the laboratory is not necessarily what it does in the human body, and the final test of every drug is in the clinical situation. Any drug may upset some patients and there is no way of telling which patient may be sensitive. Medicine like this is mere trial and error.

The homoeopath is not concerned chiefly with the laboratory tests in proving the efficacy of homoeopathic medicine since clinical experience demonstrates daily that such medicine is capable of remarkable cures. What is more the *Materia Medica* tells me on which patient I may expect a good result. Doctors new to homoeopathic medicine are finding this as they apply what they have learned from their lectures on the *Materia Medica*.

A new doctor writes—'A number of years ago, dissatisfied with the way I was practising as a GP much of my time being spent in suppressing symptoms by giving more and more expensive and generally potent and dangerous drugs, often producing disturbing side effects, I attended my first homoeopathic course in London. I now use both the conventional and homoeopathic approach to my patients' problems but use more and more homoeopathy with very good results. It seems to me, and to a number of other doctors, that the homoeopathic approach ought to be much more thought of in general practice than it is at present.

Apart from my absolutely sincere conviction that homoeopathic preparations can and often do have a powerful beneficial effect, they are completely without adverse side effects.'

Another new doctor also found a patient who was badly depressed and who responded dramatically to *Lilium tigrinum*. He referred to the first time he saw her when she was so depressed and suicidal that she might have been admitted to hospital for observation and been put on a long course of anti-depressants. It is this power in homoeo-pathic medicine which gives homoeopathy its rightful place in medicine today.

Early enthusiasm for antibiotics in treating infections has lessened because of the resistant organisms and an increasing number of patients who are hypersensitive to the drugs. Moreover, a lot of infections in the population are of viral origin, and antibiotics do not affect these. In this situation it is of inestimable value to have one's homoeopathic *Materia Medica*, from which to choose the medicine for the patients particular symptom complex. Thus we can avoid the danger which antibiotic treatment may produce, of sensi-tivity in the patient and bacterial resistance to the drug; with the additional problems which it causes of toxic effects in the body, resistance to infection in general—aggravated by vitamin deficiency—and complicated by the over-growth of fungus and rarer resistant bacteria.

Hahnemann began his special study of medicines by recording all the cases of poisoning he could find in the medical literature of the time; only after some years of this investigation did he turn his attention to drug provings. The study of poisons and provings may constitute a meeting point between homoeopathy and orthodox medicine. Drugs which have been chosen for a proving in London since 1945 have been substances which have been extensively proved, chemically, physically and biologically by researchers in other fields. This has thrown light on the particular drugs and their effects. In studying the nature of healing agents it has been part of the homoeopathic approach to take all the new discoveries into consideration.

In the past thirty years there has been a renewal of provings undertaken by homoeopathic doctors. In 1965 the late Dr Raeside conducted a proving of *Colchicum autumnale* (the autumn crocus) with seventeen provers. This work began in the autumn using the 30th potency. Many symptoms were produced, mostly in the first trial when the plant was in flower. He used a 6x potency the first time and a 6c the third:

> Some of the provers felt very alert during the first few days, but this was followed by mental lethargy, irritability, tiredness and depression. There were various head symptoms—vertigo, faintness, headaches, frontal or on the left temple, or persistent hammering head pains, heavy head, tired eyes. Eyelids sore and red. Ulcers in mouth and dry throat. Many digestive symptoms. Loss of appetite and nausea improved by eating. Heartburn—acidity of stomach. Burning pains in abdomen worse in the morning. Rumbling and fullness. Empty feeling. Palpitations and irregular heart felt by about half the provers. Stiff, aching pain in the back. Backache and stiff neck. Stiff shoulders, pain right shoulder, hand or left arm. Pains in upper arms—worse on movement. Tingling. Cold hands. Pain left leg and thigh—possibly left knee. Twitching or numbness right foot. Cold numb feet. Skin sensitive, and may be hot and burning with no sweating. *Pruritis ani.* Restless sleep—silly

dreams. Cannot sleep on right side. General fatigue. Weak and trembling.

Twelve provers out of seventeen experienced diarrhoea. Nine had frontal headaches, eight had pains in the shoulder and small joints of the hands, and six suffered from vertigo and faintness.

In recent provings on *Rauwolfia* (a member of the *Apocynaceae* plants from India) the 6c and 30th potencies were used. The recordings were as follows:

Weariness on violent exertion. Irritable and depressed—alone. Cannot be bothered—sluggish mentally, needs driving. Abrupt and most rude in attitude. Spells words wrongly, forgets where they are. Mental exhaustion. Bad headache, bursting—sore pressure in head on combing hair, as if head would float off while walking. Constriction of head like tight band. Brain feels sore, particularly in cold wind. Pressure across eyes on walking, cold hands. Eyes heavy, tired aching, burning sore edges, very sore eyelids, better for cold application. Heat and redness right ear. Dry lips—metallic taste. Skin of face dry, with pulsating throbbing tooth-ache. Nose streaming out of doors. Tight chest evening—breathless—constriction upper chest like pull from the stomach to the back on coughing. Extreme breathlessness—heart beats in throat, feels he has run miles. Thumping beat of heart climbing stairs. Sharp pain abdomen, feels hard as stone. Loose bowels—hunger ten minutes after food. Wind after food. Hunger for savouries. Thirst for cold water. Constant desire to eat. Stiffness back muscles. Stiffness left knee when going up and down stairs. Right foot frozen all evening. Sudden sharp pains anywhere, wrist, thumb, knee, aching as if strained. Burning soles of feet. Dreams of travelling, or of being killed. Irritation of skin, cracked heels. Out of world feeling. Hot flushed, sweating and sinking as if afraid. Wants to fly to open window.

Of the provers six experienced excessive drowsiness and sleepiness, four were depressed, three had diarrhoea, two suffered from anorexia, two from nausea and vomiting, two from vertigo, two had increased polyuria and one had griping pains in the abdomen.

It is interesting to note that in the provings of each of these substances there is a different picture from that of any other. Some organ or system or tissue is always selectively affected. In the case of the *Colchicum* provers it was left sided pains in the shoulder and knee, but pain in the right hand.

One can see in this list of symptoms a certain order which demonstrates the manner in which provers were asked to record their symptoms. One has not been able to improve on the order of recordings which Hahnemann suggested. But mental and head symptoms have always taken precedence. The important point is that the ordinary person proving a remedy has no knowledge of anatomy or systems of the body and will not, therefore, relate the symptoms he experiences to any idea of physiological causes. Both these remedies that I have described in provings are in use today by the orthodox doctor. *Colchicum* is still used in gout in high doses until it produces its toxic digestive symptoms. The modern pharmacologist does not really know a lot about how it works in spite of its many centuries of use in clinical practice. As homoeopaths we see patients with gout who frequently have digestive symptoms in addition, and who respond quickly to a 10m of *Colchicum*. Others, depending on the totality of symptoms, will need *Ledum*, *Arnica* or *Sulphur*. With a high uric acid level following an acute attack, Dr Compton-Burnett found that a course of *Urtica urens* in low potency brought it down and prevented further attacks.

In the provings of *Rauwolfia* some symptoms were produced which closely resembled those of high blood pressure, though the provers themselves had normal blood pressure. Their blood pressure, blood urea and urine were examined weekly during the provings. *Rauwolfia* itself has been used for blood pressure in chemical form with frequent incidence of depression as its side effect. The chemists have extracted the active principle, Reserpine, which has not shown this side effect to such a marked degree. Recently it has been noted that women taking *Rauwolfia* have a tendency to develop mammary tumours; although whether this is due to the drug or to a metabolic change associated with high blood pressure is not known. Extensive observations are now being undertaken to investigate this problem further. When the homoeopathic doctor uses *Rauwolfia* in potency he will choose it on the total picture which so often responds closely to the provings. A patient known to a homoeopathic doctor likes and uses Rautrex, which is a commercial derivative of *Rauwolfia*, for treatment for her blood pressure rather than any other known drug. She got no side effects and it kept her blood pressure in perfect control.

The situation is even more complicated in the agricultural field, where antibiotics have been used widely and often unwisely to treat sick animals. Traces of antibiotics can be passed on to people in the form of food such as milk, eggs and meat thus sensitizing allergic subjects so that should they be given the same during an infective illness in therapeutic dosage they show an allergic reaction.

In farming too, sprays are used on fruit and vegetables to kill off blights and parasites. These sprays are poisonous to man and beast and, if inhaled, can cause irreversible neurological disease. What is often forgotten is that plants concentrate these poisons in their root formation which may then be eaten by man and animal, and prove more poisonous than expected. On the continent this has been found to be true with nitrogenous fertilizers when babies become very ill after being given vegetables which had been grown in treated soil. This is also true of fluorides as well where plants concentrate fluoride to levels which are known to be toxic to human beings—reference shows that they were regarded as edible.

Physicians are finding that natural products are safer

in natural form than those chemically produced. This is true of the hormones, particularly oestrogen—and where it is necessary to advise replacement therapy in the meno-pausal phase the naturally produced oestrogen product, Premarin, is preferred to the others of the group. In Cortisone too, many side-effects are avoided if hydro-cortisone, both as an external application and when given by mouth, is used.

Another contemporary interest is in poisonous snakes and spiders which are the subject of modern chemical investi-gations to develop an antidote to the poisonous symptoms. These poisons have been known to the homoeopath for over a hundred years and have been used in the treatment of severe illness in potency. In my own experience a doctor was rung one night by another who wanted to know if he was a homoeopath, and asked him to see a child with purpura. The patient had seen a specialist from one of the teaching hospitals and was obviously dying. He had a poor blood condition altogether with a very low platelet count, and when seen he was bleeding from everywhere— the nose, mouth, bladder, bowel, and was bruised from head to foot. He was given *Crotalus horridus* (rattle snake) and he did very well indeed. His platelet count went up from a very dangerous level to nearly normal within a few days, and he began to sleep well. He was therefore, out of danger within a short time. He was sent to hospital for a blood transfusion for his consequent anaemia. The con-sultant who had seen him previously and said he was dying, pointed him out to the students as an example of spon-taneous cure which cannot be accounted for, although he knew full well he had had homoeopathic snake venom as a remedy.

The Community Physician, or district health officer who used to be concerned with and advise on infectious illness of any kind in his area is now more widely concerned in the health of the nation and in social problems such as housing, drug addiction, the care of the disabled, both young and old, where too little help is available. These problems were also the concern of Hahnemann who listed social conditions amongst the problems interfering with homoeopathic cures.

Surgery can do so much now in helping patients with structural problems. Congenital abnormalities are now often able to be corrected, the most dramatic being some valvular malformations in the heart and stenosis in the gut particularly. This is chiefly due to the advances in modern anaesthesia. Trauma from accidents makes up for a large measure of some surgeons' work and they are very competent at restoring badly injured patients to normal life. Again homoeopathy can be invaluable as an aid to prevent complications.

At all times it is obviously important to be able to teach doctors in training the part that homoeopathy can play in the various spheres of medicine. Homoeopathic doctors use all the modern techniques in the investigation of disease. This is essential in arriving at a clinical and pathological diagnosis which are not used in finding the constitutional remedy which also determines the prognosis.

The time is coming fast when homoeopathy must come into its own and be recognized on its results. So it is essential that it continues to carry out its well-tested principles. Homoeopathic provings might be carried out by the Medical Research Council to be tested in a wider sphere, if the Council were willing to establish an investigation into the experiments of Hahnemann's day.

14

Preventive Medicine

Patients who turn to homoeopathic medicine find that they are healthier in every way and look upon it in so many cases as a means of preventing colds, attacks of bronchitis and flu, injuries, car sickness or travelling difficulties. Many feel that their blood pressure is controlled, that they get less palpitations, fewer headaches and that the after-effects of old illnesses can be cleared up. They know how well they have done with their rheumatism, how they can rely on help with their hay-fever and prevent its coming on and what wonderful assistance they have had in treating their skin diseases. They regard homoeopathy as their type of medicine and choose it whenever possible because of the foresight and commonsense of the treatment.

Homoeopathy plays an important preventive role where there are children. What do people do without *Arnica* in the house? From the time that a child begins to move about it is prone to bruises, bumps and minor injuries and *Arnica* can safely be called a household remedy to relieve pain, swelling and laceration. It is also very useful in helping fractures to heal. Many surgeons have acknowledged its use in preventing post-operative complications and its help in restoring normal sleep. Its other great use is in the prevention of tissue damage after an operation and it speeds up the healing processes. For people who have to travel a great deal, especially by air and over great distances, *Arnica* will prevent mental and physical fatigue and exhaustion.

Homoeopathy in many cases and at all ages can delay or prevent surgery. All homoeopaths recognize the need for surgery and recommend it when absolutely necessary, as all doctors do. However, the homoeopath with the right remedy can prevent certain things and save surgical interference. In the treatment of boils, for instance, *Silica* or *Hepar sulph* or *Calcarea sulphurica* can be excellent remedies in making the boils discharge and clear quickly. Nowadays tonsillectomy is frequently not advised in young people. Nevertheless various forms of tonsilitis still plague children and an operation may be avoided by homoeopathic treatment. It is perfectly possible to prevent the need for an operation where the tonsils may be chronically enlarged with a history of sub-acute flare-ups of some frequency and, in most cases, where the neck glands are definitely swollen at the same time. The patient gives a definite symptom picture of a rawness in the throat, with shooting pain on attempting to swallow, as if there was a plug in the throat. The patient may choke on taking solids and will complain that the throat feels worse on empty swallowing, but all right on taking fluids. Often this patient also has a chronic enlargement of the cervical glands and a bad taste in the mouth with an amelioration from drinking. He is chilly and is typically a soft, flabby, pale patient without much stamina. He may have eruptions round the ears, with an accumulation of mucus in the nose, throat, and larynx. Generally *Baryta carbonica* will clear it up and considerably reduce the tonsils in size. There are several other remedies that reduce the size of the tonsils and clear a chronic infection. A remedy we have often found effective is *Hepar sulph* where one frequently meets a recurrent sore throat and the patient complains of a fish-bone sensation in the throat, and altogether, has a very painful, offensive mouth, the worse for touch and swallowing; and any movement such as opening the mouth or putting out the tongue increases the pain. This patient is apt to wrap a shawl or scarf around the neck and is generally the better for warmth. He sweats profusely without relief, is very chilly, keeps well covered up and he even hates to put a hand out of bed.

Another throat remedy which can clear very quickly and possibly prevent the need for surgery is *Phytolacca*. This seems to suit the very hopeless and indifferent person whose problem is a rather acute dark red throat with swollen or oedematous uvula, who feels very ill and knocked out by the infection. He complains of severe pain on putting out his tongue, and that this pain shoots up to the ear very often. The whole throat is relieved by a cold drink and is worse for a hot drink. The mouth generally is offensive and the tongue raw, as if scalded and has a yellow coating or a yellow streak down the centre. These throat infections are often accompanied by aching in the bones and joints and often an acute back ache. The throat clears completely with this remedy; within a few days it looks normal and the inflamation does not recur.

We very seldom see cases of acute mastoid nowadays because antibiotics have killed off streptococci and other germs. But, where there is a family history of ear, nose and throat trouble there have been cases in the young where a mastoidectomy was prevented by the use of *Capsicum* 10m.

There are also all the urinary problems for which homoeopathy offers such safe and effective medicines and which prevent a continuation of the trouble or any of the complications that may arise. *Causticum* is one of the chief remedies for cystitis and is often given as a preventive to those who have a tendency to a weak bladder and may be embarking on a long bus ride. This remedy is a standby to the homoeopath, and I have often known patients who take it on long sight-seeing expeditions or functions lasting several hours. One other great use of *Causticum* is to prevent the retention of urine after an operation. This is often quickly effective and will obviate the use of a catheter. Or it can be helpful after an operation where there is acute cramp in the rectum on trying to pass water. Its use can often prevent the need for antibiotics after surgery.

Berberis can save a patient from being operated on for a kidney stone. There are various very marked symptoms which indicate the need for this medicine—a digging, sticking pain in one kidney region which is aggravated by deep pressure and which radiates from one spot, either sideways or up and down. The whole back is affected and the discomfort is accompanied by stiffness so that, if stooping, the patient finds it difficult to get up and he describes it as a tearing pain. Burning in the bladder is frequently present and this may also be radiating and is described as a violent sticking pain from the kidney down to the bladder. The urine is often pale with a transparent gelatinous sediment, or a turbid clay-like, rather copious sediment, or there may be blood in it. The patient is very chilly in the morning, but hot and sweating profusely in the afternoon. With these indications it is quite possible for a kidney stone to pass after giving *Berberis* and so prevent the need for surgery.

The widespread use of the newly discovered antibiotics in the 1950s and 1960s has been followed by an increased evidence of immunological deficiency problems in babies and young children. The health of future generations has already been jeopardized by the use of hormone therapy and X-rays in expectant mothers. Homoeopathy has a large part to play in gynaecology and obstetrics. Many patients have an unexpectedly easy confinement after taking *Caulophyllum* for a month before delivery.

In *post-partum* complaints the homoeopathic remedies are often very useful. Should the new mother run a temperature and generally feel very unwell we might prescribe *Lachesis* or the patient's constitutional drug to prevent haemorrhage or some other complication.

Virus infections in early pregnancy can generally be harmful, but homoeopathic medicine can prevent complication both in the mother and the infant. As in all cases it is the individual patient and her symptoms which will determine the course of treatment because it is essential to prevent abnormal formations in a rapidly growing foetus. Homoeopathy comes into its own again here in relieving the patient without harming the infant.

Another field of preventive medicine can be seen in the allaying of hay-fever and allergies in general. People who have been treated for hay-fever can very often ward off attacks by taking a remedy that has helped them early enough. Many patients have learned when to start their individual remedy, such as *Phleum pratense*, made from timothy grass, which will prevent the trouble coming on when the grass is first cut, or from the pollen for those who know their particular sensitivity and can be given a remedy made from a mixture of pollens. It has also been found that a patient's constitutional remedy will also prevent an outbreak of their symptoms of hay-fever.

The onset of bronchitis can frequently be prevented. Again and again in a busy homoeopathic general practice one gives the constitutional remedy to prevent the patient from getting his usual bronchitis. Of these *Calcarea carbonica* in the autumn will often give a patient a winter free of colds. *Sulphur* can be another great cold preventive in the typical hot, untidy 'Sulphur patient'. In the thin, narrow-chested, very bright young adult *Phosphorus* is a remedy to think of in preventing the usual cold. One of the results in our practice was in a man of over seventy who had chronic emphysema and a hypertrophied left ventricle in his heart. He used to get bad chest pains in the morning within the first hour of waking. While he was dressing he would put half a tablet of nitroglycerine under his tongue. His wife said, that by then he looked blue and was fighting for breath. In fact, she said, it was more a gasping than a breathing. He then would take a dose of *Laurocerasus* 6. He travelled to the city by train and had a five minute walk to his office. Upon arrival he would often appear so blue and breathless that his colleagues thought he was going to die. He then took his second dose of *Laurocerasus* and within half an hour was better and quite able to do the work of the day. Originally he had been taken by his homoeopathic doctor to a heart specialist who had his chest X-rayed. His heart was seen to be grossly enlarged and his lungs showed signs of extensive emphysema. Four years later he went to see the same specialist who at first had not expected him to live who then remarked that his chest was much better than it had been before. *Laurocerasus* was his great standby for the rest of his life; it prevented further congestion and permitted him to breathe more freely.

Another field where homoeopathy is used a great deal is in gastro-intestinal troubles, where it can prevent so many problems. With so much travelling abroad nowadays people can pick up exotic germs which usually upset the bowel. In investigating diarrhoea the experts so often cannot find any of the dysenteries or traces of parasites. Here our homoeopathic bowel remedies come in: *Dysentery Co.*, *Morgan* or one of the other nosodes can prevent and clear the trouble completely. *Acidum phosphoricum* and *Arsenicum* are both very useful in the hospital nursery where one sometimes encounters epidemic diarrhoea caused by one of the pathogenic *Escherichia coli*. Nurseries sometimes have to be closed for weeks to get rid of these organisms when the infants suffer a lot from diarrhoea. The two remedies can often cut short an attack. The other children can be prevented from becoming affected, as well as the staff and helpers by a few doses of the *Escherichia coli* nosode. The fact that we have this trouble is so often due to transference of resistance from another organism to the *Escherichia coli* and therefore the failure of treatment because of the widespread use of antibiotics in man and animal.

In treating patients with symptom complexes which indicate the imminent onset of a disorder, homoeopathy prevents the development of ulcers and their complications. One has constantly found this oneself; for example, in the 'lean and livery' young man who is worried about business and suffers greatly from anticipation, who cannot be kept waiting for his lunch because he feels terrible, whose mind is so active that he cannot relax at night when he goes to bed, and who sleeps very late—the patient who needs *Lycopodium*. This stabilizes his whole make-up and prevents the development of duodenal ulcer as a result of business or family worries. I have found that they may not need anything further, particularly if they are young when first seen. On the other hand, stresses recur and may again put the organism out of balance. This recurrence of the similar symptoms usually indicates a need for a repeat of the same medicine, their constitutional remedy. This illustrates the ability of homoeopathic medicine to balance the whole patient facing recurrent stress and will prevent pathological changes. Preventive medicine enables the body's self-regulating mechanism to respond to a stress situation without recourse to drugs.

The principle of preventive medicine is apparent when one considers vaccination. In vaccinating a person against small-pox one produces an isolated vesicle which is the outward sign that the lymphocytes of the body have recognized the challenge of the small-pox organism. This recognition is permanent and later in life, if the person should be in contact with the disease, the antibodies in the system will kill it off before infection can occur. This is preventive medicine in its most orthodox meaning. We see it also in every other immunological procedure.

Going back to Hahnemann's use of *Belladonna* in preventing scarlet fever: it has *not* been shown that this remedy increases the specific immune response to the streptococcus of the infection, but in the clinical situation Hahnemann realized that patients who had had *Belladonna* did not contract scarlet fever.

The same is true of the homoeopathic oral 'flu vaccine. Clinical experience proves that protection is given in individuals, yet there is no increase of any antibodies to the influenza virus. Modern virology explains this by stating that we are not measuring the correct parameter of immunity. One cannot ignore clinical observations but we have no way of measuring true reasons—it just works. The results, therefore, of homoeopathy in preventive medicine are justifiably based on experience rather than experiment.

It is widely acknowledged that hygienic measures in public health which were advocated by Hahnemann did a lot to prevent epidemic diseases before the introduction of widespread immunization. The epidemic of polio in the 1950s had already started to abate before the effect of the use of Salk vaccine could be verified. The use of oral Sabin vaccine has made immunization against polio safe, and one usually recommends it. The medical profession generally recognizes that there are always problems with all the other immunizations. Every doctor advises on what he thinks is the best combination of immunization in the particular family circumstance. With the use of homoeopathic medicine some of the possible problems related to immunization can be prevented.

The concept of immunization against disease and epidemic is in theory a good thing; however in practice it raises problems. Homoeopathic physicians can offer effective treatment for the naturally occurring diseases such as whooping cough and measles so that one of the strong reasons for advocating immunization is removed, and quite rightly. We must be careful not to take a good thing too far. Preventive medicine should not go so far as to eliminate the production of the antibodies against a disease, because when the immunity has been removed, the introduction of a virus to a community may result in fatality. Such cases have been observed in the Arctic when the accidental introduction of the measles virus proved fatal to so many Esquimo Indians.

In considering patients from babyhood, through childhood and adolescence one recognizes the importance of mental and physical growth. This observation helps us to acquire an understanding of the value of building up resistance to infection in general so that, as an adult, one is not subject to constant illness. The immune system of the body responds to each challenge by germ or virus and develops specific resistance which may be of long or short duration. The infectious diseases themselves play a part in the development of the child and the naturally produced immunity is so much more valuable than that produced by injections. Furthermore side effects of convulsions, say after an inoculation against whooping cough, cannot occur if the immunity is built in naturally. One of the values of having an infectious disease can be seen in the clearing up of eczema after an attack of measles, as Hahnemann described in his *Organon*. A perfect example of this was in a recent case of a baby boy with severe eczema and food intolerance. He was admitted to a children's hospital for investigation at a time when there were a number of cases of measles. The baby contracted the disease and after the rash subsided his eczema disappeared completely and his health improved enormously.

The importance of the immune system in the body in preventing many illnesses has become more and more evident since the use of cortisone and immuno-suppressive therapy in patients who have had kidney transplants. These patients may have been kept alive but, according to statistics, some have developed cancer more easily. It is known now that the body has its own built-in mechanism against cancer cells and many ways are now being used to stimulate this resistance in a general fight against malignancy. Looking at cancer as a general, rather than an organ disease is now more common in both medical and surgical departments. Considering the patient as a whole is what the homoeopath has always aimed at, and he is very pleased to see this being considered in the different departments of medicine in hospitals and particularly in general practice.

The importance of trace elements is nearly inestimable in preventive medicine. One of the first to be found as essential to good health was vitamin C in fresh fruit and vegetables. During the First World War vitamin D found in dairy products was used to prevent the recurrence of rickets. It was most enthusiastically added to baby foods without any idea that it might have some side effects; as a result many children became victims of kidney complaints through over usage. At the same time it was found that soldiers in the overseas armies were developing skin trouble to an alarming extent and that some fell victim to dementia. The diets were examined and were found lacking in sufficient vitamin B which will bring on Beri beri.

It is difficult to demonstrate marginal deficiency of

specific vitamins, but clinical practice has shown that certain patients improve and put on weight after being given *Arnica* and many doctors follow on in the tradition of their elders and use cytamen injections to improve well being in the elderly, who may not in fact show a low B_{12} blood level. Protein malnutrition is often associated with vitamin B deficiencies and the World Health Organization is investigating the problem. In countries where the population is more susceptible to infections and all sorts of diseases, homoeopathy can play its part. But the important thing is to prevent the malnutrition which is so common in countries like India and Pakistan where homoeopathy is widely practised.

Biologists have been investigating the importance of many trace elements in the body and have found that in some animals exceptionally small quantities are essential for some of the metabolic processes. This has been discussed at a World Conference, and these studies, although still in their infancy, point to the importance of micro-elements in the body, micro-elements which were previously considered unimportant. Some of these trace elements are used as homoeopathic remedies, and the clinical picture they present is in some cases similar to that of the deficiency artificially produced in the laboratory animal. The homoeopathic potency stimulates a return to normal although we cannot yet explain it. There is here a wide-open field for scientific investigation which might lead to a greater understanding of how homoeopathic treatment works.

In the 1930s, referred to as the first Golden Era of the discovery of trace elements, the nutritional significance of copper, zinc, manganese and cobalt were discovered. With increasing advances in analytical techniques the importance of such elements has been emphasised. In certain areas of the Middle East where there is a high incidence of dwarfism among men, it was found that there is a marked deficiency of zinc in their diet. The other discovery is the importance of cadmium in cases of hypertension. Chromium has been recently discovered to improve glucose tolerance in elderly diabetics. The mode of action of the trace element is unknown. In 1963 Professor Underwood wrote from Australia: 'embarrassingly little is yet known of the precise metabolic roles of the trace elements'.

Another important realm in preventive medicine is in avoiding the after-effects of some infection. We commonly see patients who have never been well since their infectious disease either in childhood or as adults. In most of these cases the nosode is required before they will finally clear up. If they are seen during their acute illness any remedy may be needed; but if symptoms still hang on, and the patient does not completely recover, one must think again of the nosode related to that particular disease. Until recently it was not known what caused glandular fever, but now a virus, called the E.B. virus has been isolated. This is one of the diseases which tends to hang on. A few years ago a homoeopathic doctor seeing a patient in the acute phase took a sample of his blood and tested it for the virus. The Paul Bunnell test was strongly positive and the blood sample was sent to the homoeopathic chemist to have a potency run up. This is now available as a glandular fever nosode fulfilling the criteria of Hahnemann's original nosode that the disease product rather than the virus itself forms the basis of the medicine which can be used.

A great many of the extracts used in homoeopathic remedies have been proved; others have been used clinically and the results collected and recorded. This has given many extra symptoms at times, and a repetition of these symptoms has been added to the general clinical picture of the remedy so that clinical provings have resulted in a very full picture on which to prescribe.

The fact that a trituration is made of a whole plant gives enormous possibilities for the preparation of homoeopathic remedies to be used for world health. It is so much safer to deal with a whole than some particular part in the preparation of the drug. Raw material is indigenous, easily available and easily rendered into suitable medicines. Given sufficient warning of probable disaster in a developing area, it would be possible to avoid epidemics by training the doctors to use the material on hand on both humans and animals and thus avoid an economic world crisis.

In certain situations what may appear to be a cure of an epidemic state may well alleviate a present outbreak temporarily, but in the end may precipitate a disaster. It is rather like the situation in the USA and Egypt when it was thought that hydroelectric dams were the solution to land reclamation and fertilization. In the end, after not too many years it was found that, far from helping the people, thousands of acres of arable land had been destroyed through increased salination. Again, intensive farming seemed to be a solution, but has now proved to have taken so much of the goodness out of the soil, as well as destroying the life of insects and worms in the ground, that it is a destructive process and may well ruin the prospects of good crops for future generations.

So in world health terms, and especially in the poorer countries, we can also help to prove that the relief of a symptom will not result in another symptom. Which is what happened in the instance of thalidomide. This could not happen in homoeopathic treatments, as has been proved by experimentation over the years. It is also recognized that the side effects of antibiotics are decreasing resistance to some household diseases, such as whooping cough and measles. In fact, it has recently been suggested that, after careful investigation, the measles inoculation may actually increase the incidence of disseminated sclerosis.

Homoeopathy has proved beneficial for so many years by careful testing on people and clinical results. A lot of medicines have originated in what are known as the under-developed countries. *Curare* found in South America, was developed from the poison of a plant and used on arrow heads. But it is also used in the relief of certain forms of muscular tension. *Arnica montana* leaves have been chewed by mountaineers to give them strength in climbing. *Colchicum autumnalis* has been used for 2000 years for gouty and rheumatic complaints. Working on homoeopathic prin-ciples this has been proved and reproved countless times, yet the modern chemist still does not know how it acts to help gout. Nettles—*Urtica urens*—have been known and used for burns, urticaria and other complaints.

There is a world map of indigenous plants so that we can pick out what is available to be used on homoeopathic principles. The present use of herbs has been a long-standing tradition; such things as 'bush tea' are well known for their healing properties. Provings have been done on a large number of herbs of known repute.

Local remedies are so often close to hand for local diseases. One has only to think of dock for stinging nettles. In some areas in the Balkans and Asia Minor there are records of longevity and in every instance there have been recorded traces of arsenic in the diet.

Much training and experiment has to be done in the developing countries to enable them to treat indigenous diseases with indigenous cures. Local medicines are more effective and longer lasting in curative powers for local outbreaks of disease. The needs in one country are not necessarily the same for every other country. By educating and encouraging the people of the developing world to seek out by experimentation and provings their own natural remedies a great burden would be lifted from them and those countries which, in times of emergency, have had to come to their assistance.

The developing countries have a prospect of hope and independence if they were to work out such a programme. If they are encouraged to adapt their native gifts to their native requirements they may be closer to medical and economic independence. But the wholesale destruction of the forests of the Amazon, where so many natural sources of medicine will be lost, is surely one of the great tragedies of our time and for the future health of the world.

What a tremendous challenge homoeopathy must face for the health of the nations. The remedies are there: all that is needed is enough doctors who are willing to train in the concept of healing, who will accept the challenge to apply what has been put into the world to alleviate human suffering.

15

The Homoeopathic Bouquet

In a few instances the specific plant was not available for the bouquet and so a substitute plant of the same species was used.

1. Dog rose (*Rosa canina*)—
Tincture of ripe fruits. It was used in ancient times as a remedy for urinary difficulties and is still used for dysuria and affections of the bladder. Dr Compton-Burnett confirmed this to some extent. A proving which he carried out produced only a somewhat marked increase of urine flow.

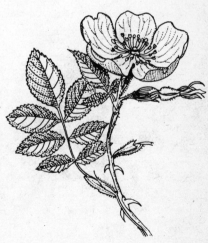

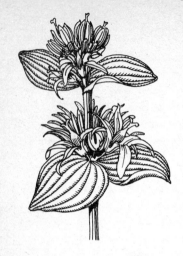

2. Gentian

Of which the *Gentiana lutea* is used.

It is well known as a tonic in ordinary medicine. In homoeopathy the symptoms have been noticed most markedly in the alimentary sphere, so that one meets 'ravenous hunger' as well as 'diminished appetite'. It has some claim therefore to be a 'positive tonic' as it may cause increased appetite in the healthy.

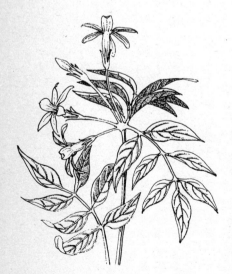

3. White Jasmine
(*Jasminum officinale*)

Tincture of red berries.

It has only been recorded on very slight knowledge of its provings in a boy who ate the red berries which produced a comatose state, vomiting, convulsions, and finally tetanus. It has been used in the treatment of tetanus and convulsions on occasions.

5. Primrose (*Primula vulgaris*)

This is sometimes very good in the case of dropsy.

6. St John's wort (*Hypericum*)

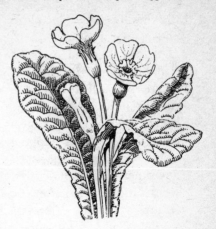

The tincture is made of the whole fresh plant.

This remedy is used extensively by homoeopaths. The leaves of various species of *Hypericum* are sprinkled with pellucid dots and black glands which contain an essential oil. The *Hypericum perforatum* is the most conspicuous for its oil, and in consequence, is used chiefly as a remedy for wounds or perforations of the integuments and from olden times the leaves were applied to flesh wounds. They were called 'Tutsan' (*toute saine*). The word *Hypericum* means 'sub-heather' indicating its manifest relationship to the heaths. *Hypericum* underwent a very intensive proving, and brings out the 'relation of the drug to wounds and their consequences, and its application to maladies of other kinds'— such as a 'fuzzy' feeling on

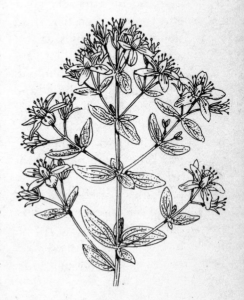

the hands, shaking, pains and a paralytic weakness. *Hypericum* is found to be of signal service in wounds where the affected part is rich in nerves, such as the brain, spine, coccyx, finger-ends, wounds from stepping on nails or sharp objects, or any other kind of punctured wound. The characteristic feature of the *Hypericum* wound is that it is very sensitive to touch.

Hypericum can also be very useful in nervous depression following wounding, and the effects of shock or fright, and it is also used to very good effect for ulceration and sloughing of wounds. It will also be found useful for very painful corns and bunions. The patient is chilly and worse for damp or cold air and fog. There are homoeopathic preparations of *Hypericum* oil and ointment which are particularly useful in applying to bed-sores, and for applications to wounds, cuts and abrasions. *Hypericum* can also be used as a compress and is found to be very soothing.

7. Yellow Jasmine (*Gelsemium*)

Tincture of bark of the root.

This is a continuously used homoeopathic remedy. It belongs to the same order of plants as *Nux vomica* and *Curare*.

Patients needing this remedy manifest a number of well-marked and clearly characterized symptoms met with in everyday practice. This has given it a place among the polycrests of homoeopathy. Like its botanical relatives, *Gelsemium* is a great paralyzer. The mind is sluggish, the whole muscular system is relaxed. The limbs feel almost too heavy to move. Functional paralyses is shown on some features of the headaches. They are accompanied by blurring of the sight, and relieved by a copious discharge of watery urine. The mental prostration is typified in 'funk' as before for instance, an examination of some kind, stage-fright, effects of bad nerves, and is often accompanied by drooping eyelids—alcoholic stimulants relieve the complaint where *Gelsemium* is useful. It is an excellent remedy for neuralgic headaches beginning at the top of the spine and extending over the head causing a bursting pain in the head and eyeballs accompanied by nausea, vomiting, cold sweat and cold feet. When less acute, there is a great heaviness in the head relieved by profuse micturition. A heavy dull appearance to the patient, flushed and hot to the touch. The tongue is coated, yellowish white with foetid breath and a very bad taste. There is often a dry, burning throat with hoarseness. There is usually some stomach discomfort, and a feeling of emptiness in the stomach, with a weakness there and in the bowels. Alternatively, there may be fulness and oppression in the stomach, and there is a lot of 'rumbling' and discomfort in the abdomen with a sudden, spasmodic pain which leaves a sensation of contraction afterwards. The

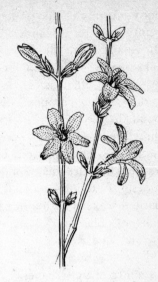

throat is frequently weak, with difficulty in swallowing at times, and often accompanied by a hoarseness and dryness with a dry cough and soreness of the chest and fluent coryza. There may be irregular heart beats and palpitation and occasionally a feeling that the heart might stop beating if the patient moves. There is frequently trembling in all the limbs and deep-seated, dull aching in the muscles, and the gait is unsteady in consequence. There is hyperaesthesia with excessive irritability of mind and body. At night the patient complains of wandering rheumatic pain. He may be very sleepy and sleep long but more often is drowsy and cannot compose his mind to sleep. The sleep, therefore, when it does come, is accompanied by unpleasant dreams, sometimes of dying—and the patient wakens with a headache, or colic.

8. Red Root
(*Ceanothus*)

Tincture of fresh leaves.

Dr Compton-Burnett following Dr Hale is our chief authority for *Ceanothus*. It

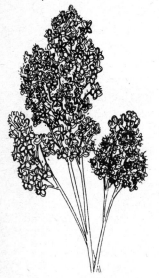

was proved in 1900 but it had already been used extensively on its definite clinical symptoms. It is a spleen remedy *par excellence*, deep seated pain in the left hypochondrium, pain and fullness in the left side. The patient is very chilly—principally down the back—worse in cold weather, and wants to sit over a fire if possible. There is often a headache with the spleen symptoms and sometimes acute diarrhoea. Those who proved *Ceanothus* got quite severe symptoms. The patients are depressed, and feel they will not be fit to work. They are chilly, have no appetite, and show a 'don't care' attitude all the time.

9. Cyclamen
(*C. neapolitanum*)

Tincture of the root in the spring.

This remedy is analogous to *Pulsatilla*, the main difference being that it is no better for open air. It is especially useful for affections of the uterus and appendages.

It is suited to the phleg-
matic temperament. The
type of patient who is disinclined to work, and easily
fatigued and who complains
of flickering before the eyes
and a tendency to squint. It
can therefore be very useful in cases of amblyopia,
diplopia and myopia. There
is also a tendency to
digestive disturbance and
the saliva has a salty taste
which is conveyed to all the
food eaten. The appetite is
poor, and there is often
aversion to bread, and many
other ordinary foods. The
patient is inclined to vomit
in the morning, and hic-
cough can be very troublesome. They become morose
with sleepiness and lassi-
tude, and that was a picture
which was particularly
marked in most of the provings.

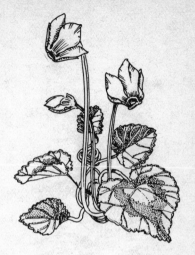

10. Sage (*Salvia*)
Tincture of fresh leaves and
blossom tips.

This is common sage, and
an 1897 medical publication
mentions its use as a gargle
and mouthwash in sore
throats and affections of the

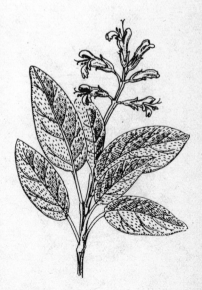

gums. It has also been found to be very useful for the tickling coughs of consumptives given as 10–20 drops of the tincture in a tablespoonful of water.

12. Rosemary
(Rosmarinus officinalis)

Tincture of the whole plant.

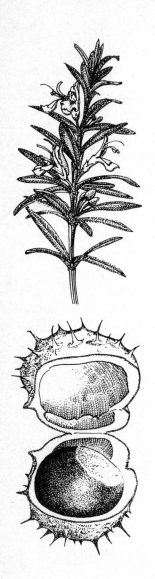

Oil of Rosemary has a long-standing reputation as a remedy for baldness, headache and flagging mental powers. Hence it has been called 'Herb of Memory', as Ophelia says in Shakespeare's *Hamlet* 'There's Rosemary for remembrance . . .'

14. Horse-chestnut
(Aesculus hippocastanum)

Tincture of ripe kernel.

This is one of the great pile remedies. The haemorrhoids are veined and bleeding and when they bleed the pain is eased. In some districts it was popular as a custom, to carry a chestnut in the pocket as a preventive. The haemorrhoids are accompanied by a feeling of dryness in the rectum as if little sticks or splinters were sticking in the mucous membranes with weak feelings on the sacro iliac joints as if the legs would give way. General aching in the lumbar and stiffness of the back.

18. Iris (*Iris foetidissima*)

The medicine is made from a tincture of the root.

Used for burning pains in the mouth and throat not relieved by cold water or anything else. A pain in the right groin. The patient feels light-headed and staggers when trying to walk. There is a great weight on vertex when pain in the stomach occurs.

19. Fools' parsley (*Aethusa cynapium*)

Tincture of whole flowering plant.

The symptoms of this herb as a remedy are particularly well known, and extremes in symptoms is one noteworthy point about its action—violent convulsions, violent pains, violent deli-

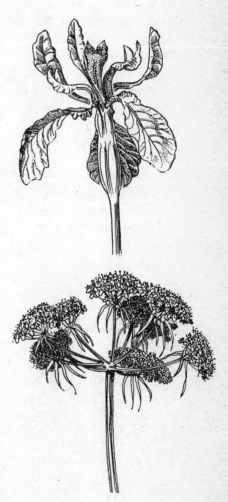

rium, violent vomiting. Although sometimes, between bouts, there may be somnolence and prostration.

Fools' parsley is not so named for nothing! It is indeed, a medicine for 'fools'. The patient has an inability to fix his or her attention or to think clearly. It is used in cases of idiocy, hallucinations, delirium, where the patient sees cats and dogs, wants to jump out of the window or out of bed, and is irritable—especially out of doors in the open air. The mental symptoms peculiar to children and sometimes to adults are great

anguish with crying, and as the illness progresses these symptoms increase, and dosage may intervene.

Another marked symptom of this remedy is the intolerance of milk, and a child may vomit in any event, but particularly with milk, and is left so exhausted that he falls asleep after vomiting. The child wakes hungry, eats, and vomits again, therefore, hunger after vomiting is a key note of the remedy.

Adults can also get a burning discomfort in the stomach which gets distended and very sensitive, and there may be a herpetic eruption on the tip of the nose, and, with the stomach symptoms, a great expression of anxiety and pain.

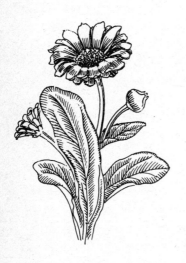

20. Marigold
(*Calendula*)

Tincture of leaves and flowers.

Calendula belongs to the same family as the other injury remedies—*Arnica* and *Bellis perennis* and is es-

pecially indicated in lacerated or suppurating wounds
and it is known to restore
the vitality of the injured
part making it impregnable
against putrefaction and is
therefore very safe and very
suitable in injury where the
skin is broken. Jahr, one of
Hahnemann's pupils who
was in Paris during the
Coup d'état of 1848, treated a
number of gun-shot wound
cases with *Calendula* and
saved a number of limbs. In
some cases of carbuncle, it
acts very quickly 'stopping
pain and fever.' It is frequently used as a hot compress and gives great comfort where there is inflammation and redness with
great deal of discomfort. It
is an excellent haemostatic
in tooth extractions and is
most valuable in mouths
with unhealthy gums, where
drops in a teacup full of hot
water tone up the gums
after massaging gently towards the teeth. The patient
needing *Calendula* as an internal remedy is extremely
sensitive to cold air particularly in cloudy weather and

it is sometimes useful as the
first remedy to be given in a
lacerated head injury.

21. Valerian
(*Valeriana*)
Tincture of fresh root.

This was proved by
Hahnemann himself and
Stapf and Franz. When
Franz wrote it was the
fashion amongst ladies of
Germany to take valerian
almost as frequently as
coffee, and to this practice
he attributed much of the
nervous suffering then
present. Franz also recorded
many of the symptoms on
taking *Valeriana*:

1. An acceleration of pulse
   and congestion of the
   head.
2. The symptoms of the
   upper and lower limbs
   alternate frequently.
3. Symptoms due to *Valeriana* are worse at noon and
   in the early afternoon
   and hours before mid-
   night.
4. *Valeriana* causes various
   kinds of darting, tearing
   pains which come and

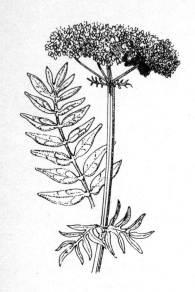

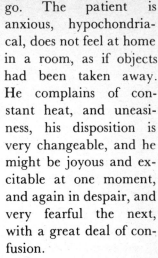

go. The patient is anxious, hypochondriacal, does not feel at home in a room, as if objects had been taken away. He complains of constant heat, and uneasiness, his disposition is very changeable, and he might be joyous and excitable at one moment, and again in despair, and very fearful the next, with a great deal of confusion.

In nervous patients *Valeriana* is known to calm them. It abates the excitement of the circulation, promotes sleep, and induces a sensation of quietude and comfort. It is also a very useful remedy in complaints involving the *tendo-achilles*.

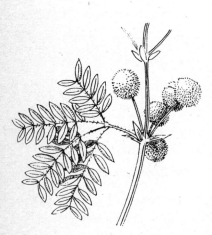

22. Mimosa (*Acacia*)
Tincture of the leaves.

The most noteable symptoms of this remedy are lancinations in the back and limbs and swelling and redness of the left ankle with tension and shooting pains.

24. Laurarticus
     (*Laurocerasus*)
    Lauristinus
     (*Viburnum tinus*)

The symptoms are a gasping
for breath, and the patient
tends to place the hand to
the heart as if there is some
trouble thereabouts. Hurry-
ing will make the patient
completely breathless.

The pupils may also be
dilated unequally.

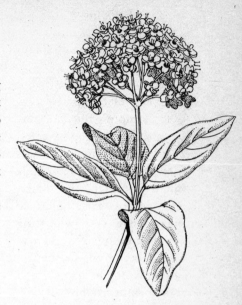

31. Snowberry
     (*Symphoricarpus*
     (*racemosus*)

Tincture of fresh ripe berries.

  Symptoms are indiffer-
ence to food, heaving
nausea, continuous vomit-
ing or violent retching. It
was used a great deal in the
old days, interest was revived with *New, Old and Forgotten Remedies* by E. T.
Moffat.

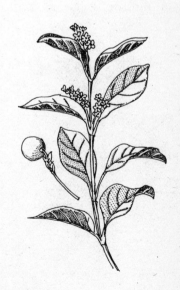

35. Stinging Nettle
(*Urtica urens*)

Tincture of the fresh plant or flower used.

Its use in gravel and urinary infections is very old. Compton-Burnett may be said to have rediscovered *Urtica* as a remedy. It was used in antiquity against inflammation of the uvula, and was a great help in pneumonia, whooping cough and pleurisy. It was also considered to be an antidote to hemlock, poisoned mushrooms, quicksilver, henbane, serpent bites and scorpions. Dr Cooper, an illustrious homoeopath,

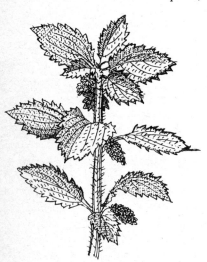

practising in the last century said that a bundle of nettles applied to a rheumatic joint or part has 'long been a favourite country remedy'. Dr Compton-Burnett used it for spleen affections and then realised that it was a great remedy for gout. He used to order 5 drops of the tincture in a wineglass of quite warm water every two or three hours, and under its action the urine became more plentiful, dark, and full of uric acid. Dr Compton-Burnett reported that he had discovered its fever-action because one of his patients was cured of ague by drinking nettle tea on the advice of her charwoman, and it became his sheet-anchor in treating the fevers of East India, Burma and Siam. It is one of the best remedies for burns of the first degree, scalds used locally and given internally. It has an antidotal quality when treating snake-bites, and it has been recorded, and claimed to be a specific for bee-stings. Symptoms calling for *Urtica* are seasonal and have been known to return each year.

36. *Clematis*

Tincture of leaves and stems.

It is a useful remedy for pimples on the face or about the ears and hair line with small discharging crusts on the scalp, gonorrhoea, headache, rheumatism and stricture of the urethra. In this last symptom it displays special modalities on which one prescribes, the flow of urine is by fits and starts or the patient has to wait a long time before being able to pass water. The urine is turbid and milky or dark and secretion is diminished. It is very difficult to empty the bladder completely. It has one very useful peculiar symptom—the patient fears to be alone yet dreads company.

37. Spindle berry
(*Euonymus*)

Trituration of dried seeds or tincture of fresh seeds.

The group to which this plant belongs is the *Celastracea* and is closely related to *Rhamnaceae* which in-

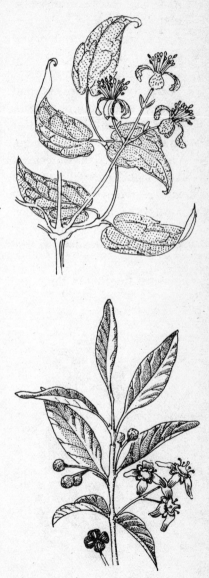

clude the purgative *Cascara sagrada*—in a poisonous dose *Euonymus* can cause acute abdominal pain and diarrhoea, collapse, and even death, but it has been used successfully for enlargement of the liver, biliousness, bad taste, coated tongue, constipation, and severe pains in the back such as lumbago, cutting pains in the cheek bones and even the tongue with violent shivering, a chill over the whole body, and often, an eruption or small dry pustules on the skin with sometimes a general tingling of the skin.

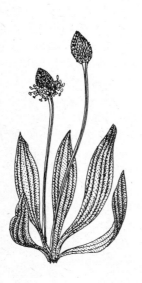

39. Plantain, or Ribwort (*Plantago*)

Plantago has a wide reputation in medicine from antiquity and homeopathy revived this reputation. In 1640 in a book called *Theatre of Plants* John Parkinson wrote, 'the root taken fresh out of the ground, washed and gently scraped with a knife then put into the ear, cures toothache like a charm'. In domestic practice it was often used in all infections of the skin, with irritation, pain from heat, the bruised leaves being applied to the part. In neuralgic conditions where the suffering part can be reached *Plantago* may be painted on with signal relief very often. Painting the gum will relieve toothache very quickly—toothache with earache, and toothache with salivation are leading symptoms.

41. Arbor Vitae (*Thuja occidentalis*)

Remedy prepared from fresh green twigs.

It was introduced to

France from Canada in the reign of Francis I. (16th Century) and spread throughout Europe. Its native habitat is not without importance in relation to therapeutics as it loves the swamps. *Thuja* was one of Hahnemann's discoveries and like most of the remedies of his *Materia medica*, had been known, in a fashion, before his time, but the therapeutic qualities of *Thuja* were not known until Hahnemann himself proved it. He found in this substance an antidote to the constitutional disease resulting from the after effect of gonorrhoea and having as its most characteristic manifestation excrescences like warts, or soft spongy-like papillomata, or highly wrinkled growths, bleeding readily, moist and with an unpleasant secretion.

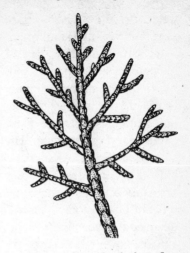

Thuja symptoms frequently occur at night. The patient may then develop symptoms of confusion or thoughts which he cannot get rid of. There will often be pain in the head, and he is often disturbed by frequent dreams, and they also describe 'floating stripes'. A keynote of *Thuja* is frequent micturition accompanying pains, and it is at times needed for enuresis. Boeninghausen of USA found *Thuja* both preventive and curative in an epidemic of smallpox. It aborted the process and prevented pitting. These facts open up another great branch of *Thuja* homoeopathicity—its anti-vaccinal action. Dr. Compton-Burnett wrote a booklet *Vaccinosis and its cure by Thuja*—by vaccinosis, he meant the disease known as vaccinia which was the result of vaccination plus that profound and often long-lasting morbid constitutional state engendered by the vaccination vaccine virus. *Thuja* is one of the best remedies for these vaccination after effects. Dr Compton-Burnett was probably the first to realize that a number of patients date their ill-health to a so called unsuccessful vaccination or a very severe vaccination reaction, and this homoeopathic doctors have experienced and confirmed ever since. *Thuja* is frequently used in this type of history in a patient, and is in daily use in most homoeopathic practices for these different complaints.

Thuja has a further relationship to more serious new growths and even malignant tumours have yielded to it. More particularly polypi or fibromata or papillomata that are the result of chronic irritation by discharges will find a remedy in *Thuja*. The patient will constantly complain of cold damp weather.

42. Christmas Rose
(*Helleborus niger*)

The juice of the fresh root mixed with equal parts of alcohol.

It is chiefly used homoeopathically for a kind of stupor when the patient does not see anything fully, although the sight is unimpaired, and does not pay attention to anything. Although his hearing is perfectly sound he does not hear anything clearly either. In this state the patient sounds very confused and answers very slowly. He may go onto actual inflammatory states of the meninges. He complains of feeling dull and stupid in the head—it was known in ancient times as a remedy for dropsy, where 'the forehead is wrinkled, there are automatic movements of one leg or arm while the other appears paralyzed. The head rolls from side to side and the patient often screams. There is greedy drinking of water and a chewing motion of the jaws, and the urine is scanty or suppressed, sometimes with a sediment like coffee grounds'. (Clarke's *Dictionary of Homoeopathy*).

Dullness and heaviness of the head are a marked feature in those needing this remedy. There is always a condition of extreme anxiety; vertigo with a sensation of reeling in the head is common with heat and fullness in the forehead. At times the headache is occipital. The patient has a pale face with distortion at times.

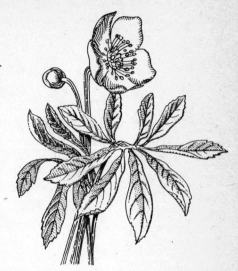

Appendices

Appendix 1
Homoeopathic
Pharmacy

Homoeopathic preparations may be described as medicaments produced in accordance with the methods described in homoeopathic *Materia Medica* or *Pharmacopoeia*, thus enabling them to be used in homoeopathic treatment. The Hahnemann process of serial dilution with succussion is considered advisable when medicines are to be produced for employment in homoeopathic treatment. The preparations are described by the use of the old latin name of the drug, substance or composition employed, followed by the conventional designation of the dilution, the following abbreviations being used:

φ for mother tinctures—the concentrated form of the medicament, T.M.

x or D (Continental) for decimal dilution,

c or cH (Continental) for centesimal dilution,

preceded or followed by a number expressing the degree of the dilution. Tablets, pills, trituration, granules, powder doses and liquid preparations all take the denomination of the dilution used.

A   *Raw Materials*

The starting material for the dilutions prepared according to the Hahnemann method may be mother tinctures, chemical products of natural or synthetic origin, biological preparations in the widest sense and any substance which may be considered of medicinal value. Many of the basic materials used in the preparation of homoeopathic medicines do not appear in standard pharmaceutical reference books.

I   MOTHER TINCTURES T.M. φ

Mother tinctures are liquid preparations resulting from the extraction of drugs of vegetable or more rarely biological origin with suitable ethanol/water mixtures.

Mother tinctures of vegetable drugs are obtained by maceration, or percolation using different strengths of ethanol or juice extraction with the juices being preserved with ethanol. Usually fresh material is used, although some dried plants or plant constituents are official. The final tincture concentration is variable and may be 1 part of drug to 1 part of final product up to 1 part to 10 parts.

Many such φ fall in the range of the 1:3 ratio. Final alcoholic strengths are approximately $33\frac{1}{3}\%$, 50%, 80% and 90%.

Mother tinctures of drugs of animal origin are also obtained by maceration in different strengths of alcohol.

Preparation of Mother Tinctures T.M. φ
The textbooks used for reference are:
The British Homoeopathic Pharmacopoeia 1882
The Homoeopathic Pharmacopoeia of the United States 1964
The American Homoeopathic Pharmacopoeia 1928
A Dictionary of Practical Materia Medica (Clarke)
and standard homoeopathic textbooks.

The most suitable method of preparation is selected from the available information. Broadly speaking the φ are divided into three main classes:

(a) *Succulent plants* yielding from 350–700ml. of juice per kg. of plant. The unfiltered expressed juice from the fresh plant is mixed with half of its volume of 95% alcohol. The finished tincture is of approximately $33\frac{1}{3}\%$ alcohol content v/v.

(b) *Fresh plants* yielding less than 350 ml. of juice per kg. of plant are comminuted and repeatedly macerated with suitable quantities of ethanol/water mixture of 87% ethanol/13% water in the proportion of 2 parts by weight of menstruum to 1 part by weight of plant. The finished φ is approximately 80% ethanol v/v.

The maceration process may utilize alcohol strengths from 60% to 87% and may be more than 1 part plant to 2 parts extractive, depending on the nature of the plant material being processed and the yield of the φ required.

(c) *Dry material*. The suitably comminuted material is percolated with 95% alcohol in the proportion of 5 parts by weight of 95% alcohol to 1 part by weight of plant. The finished φ is 90–95% alcohol.

The φ is considered to be the most concentrated stable preparation which may be economically prepared.

Collection, Preparation and Storage of Drugs

Animal substances. These should be obtained from perfect and healthy specimens and prepared in a pure and unadulterated state. They should be unmixed with any other substances and, if required to be stored prior to use in tinctures or triturations, should be protected from light, air and moisture.

Whole plants. Whole plants are collected during the flowering season in sunny weather and cleaned by careful shaking, gently rubbing or brushing, avoiding undue contact with water. Preferably, only clean specimens should be used.

Leaves and Herbs. These are collected when fully developed shortly prior to the flowering season.

Flowers. Flowers are best collected in dry weather when they are just beginning to open.

Stems. Stems are treated in the same way as leaves and are cut after the leaves have developed.

Barks. Non-resinous barks are taken from vigorous, young trees late in the autumn. Barks from resinous trees are collected at, or about the time of development of blossoms and leaves.

Woods. These are collected before the sap rises, in the early spring, from young and vigorous trees and tree-like shrubs.

Roots. Annual roots are lifted after the seeds have ripened in early autumn. Biennial roots are collected during the spring and roots of perennial plants in the second and third year prior to the development of woody fibre. Cleaning of roots, which should be as fresh as possible, is carried out avoiding the excessive use of water. They should be carefully examined to ensure the absence of dampness, mouldiness, or woody appearance.

Berries, fruits and seeds. Except in a few instances, these are all gathered when ripe. If used in a succulent state for the preparation of tinctures etc., only perfect and fresh specimens are employed. Dried fruits and seeds only may be stored in well-closed vessels. All vegetable drugs are required to be free, as far as is practicable from insects or other animal life, material or excreta. They must be free from mouldiness, abnormal odour, sliminess, discoloration or deterioration brought about through any cause.

Vehicle Standard

Vehicles such as ethanol in various strengths, milk sugar

and water used in the preparation of homoeopathic medicines should conform with the tests for identity and purity described in the British Pharmacopoeia or other accepted standard reference books.

2   BIOLOGICAL PRODUCTS

The material may be obtained from virtually any source pathological or not pathological of animal or vegetable origin etc. The dilutions are made by solution of the starting material in suitable ethanol/water mixtures and subsequent serial dilution.

3   CHEMICAL PRODUCTS OF NATURAL OR SYNTHETIC ORIGIN

This class of substances includes ores and minerals, chemical substances of organic or inorganic origin, both natural and synthetic. The substances may be insoluble in alcohol and water or of varying degrees of solubility.

B   *Potencies*

Potencies are obtained according to accepted methods designed to achieve the required degree of dilution in regular stages.

There are two methods of dilution, decimal and centesimal, depending on successive operations of reduction being in steps of 1/10 or 1/100 respectively. The number of operations thus effected determines the potency of the dilution or trituration obtained, as is shown in the table on page 218.

PREPARATION

(a) *Centesimal succussed dilutions* 1/100 ratio. Starting with the tincture or suitable liquid sample of the medicinal substance, make the succussed dilutions in progression, 1 part in 100 at each stage successively, vigorously shaking the vials at each stage—termed succussion—using the

DILUTION	CONCENTRATION		DECIMAL SCALE	CENTESIMAL SCALE	
$1/10$	10%	10^{-1}	D_1 or $1x$	$1c$ or $1cH$	$1/100$
$1/100$	1%	10^{-2}	D_2 or $2x$		
$1/1000$	$0\cdot1\%$	10^{-3}	D_3 or $3x$		
$1/10000$	$0\cdot01\%$	10^{-4}	D_4 or $4x$	$2c$ or $2cH$	$1/10000$
$1/100000$	$0\cdot001\%$	10^{-5}	D_5 or $5x$		
$1/1000000$	$0\cdot0001\%$	10^{-6}	D_6 or $6x$	$3c$	$1/1000000$
$1/10^{12}$		10^{-12}	D_{12} or $12x$	$6cH$	
		10^{-18}		$9c$	$1/10^{18}$
		10^{-24}		$12c$	$1/10^{24}$
		10^{-60}		$30c$	$1/10^{60}$

appropriate number of vials required for the degree of dilution which is to be achieved. In this manner the 6th vial will contain the 6th succussed dilution $1:10^{-12}$, the 30th vial the 30th succussed dilution $1:10^{-60}$, etc. Use neutral glass carefully cleaned vials of suitable capacity and natural unprocessed closures. There should be an air space of approximately 1/5 of the tube capacity to enable adequate mixing and shaking. Chemical substances are dissolved in suitable ethanol/water mixtures to achieve a known concentration and potentizing carried out in accordance with the described method. For medicaments available in φ it is this which is used as the starting material.

(b) *Decimal dilutions.* Proceed by the same method, but according to the decimal scale, i.e. 1/10 ratio.

(c) *Centesimal triturations.* This process is employed to render insoluble substances to a degree of fineness of subdivision which will permit solubilization in alcohol/water mixture. Triturate thoroughly and carefully in a mortar one part of the solid substance in fine powder, with a small part of the required 99 parts of lactose to be used as the diluent. Continue the trituration for 1 hour adding the rest of the diluent in aliquot parts at 20 minute intervals. Take one part of this 1st centesimal trituration and triturate as before with 99 parts of lactose to obtain the second centesimal potency; proceed in the same manner to obtain the third centesimal potency. At this stage prepare the 4c in solution with alcohol and continue as stated before for potentization by the liquid method.

C   *Pharmaceutical Forms*

There are four main types of preparation available for dispensing homoeopathic medicines, each suited to a particular type of prescription. The preparations are:

1. Powders
2. Tablets—medicated and trituration
3. Granules
4. Liquid

1   POWDERS

This is perhaps the most suitable dispensing form for the special type of homoeopathy practiced in the UK, being specially suitable for administering one or two doses of potency with intermittent placebo for any specified period. The powders are of 180mg. Lactose B.P. wrapped in high quality white paper. They are supplied numbered or un-numbered according to the need of the prescriber.

These sample prescriptions demonstrate their uses:

Numbered powders

(a) Sulphur 1m 1
    S.L. 28 mane

Powder No. 1 is medicated with Sulphur 1m.
Lactose powders 2 to 28.
One powder to be taken dry on the tongue each morning before breakfast in the order numbered (1 month's supply).

(b) Arsen. alb. 30 1–3
    S.L. 12 t.d.s.p.c.

Arsenicum album 30 in powders 1 to 3.

Lactose powders 4 to 12.

One powder to be taken dry on the tongue three times a day after meals in the order numbered (4 day's supply).

(c) Bryonia 10m 1/2   Bryonia 10m in powders 1 and 2.
    S.L. 56 n & m   Lactose powders 3 to 56.

One powder to be taken dry on the tongue each night and morning as numbered (1 month's supply).

As will be seen from these few examples many variations are possible. Powders are also of value in severe acute conditions when a relatively high rate of dosage is called for:

Not numbered powders

(d) Gelsem. 200 12 n/n   All medicated.
    2 hrly.   One powder to be taken dry on the tongue every two hours.

(e) Nux vom 30 12 n/n   All medicated.
    4 hrly.   One powder to be taken dry on the tongue every four hours.

The powders are put up in a suitable container and labelled with the necessary instructions. Possibly this dispensing form is best made up by a pharmacy with knowledge of homoeopathy and lends itself best to the treatment of the more chronic conditions; for acute states it is often better to use tablets.

2   TABLETS

(a) *Medicated tablets*. These are lactose with an added amount of pure cane sugar, 130mg. size, two for a dose. The desired potency is absorbed into the tablets and they are available in the following sizes of bottles:

7g. (gramme), approximately 50 tablets

25g. approximately 200 tablets

Any potency may be supplied, for example, the 3 or 6 or
12 or 30 or 200 etc. Specimen prescriptions would be:
Ruta 6, 7g. (or 50 tabs.) or Arnica 200 7g. (or 50 tabs.)
ii t.d.s.a.c.   ii every 15 mins. for 4 doses,
                                       then two hourly for 4 doses.
 or Belladonna 30 7g. tabs. ii hourly for 6 doses, then
                            t.d.s. for 2 days.
The tablet form may be preferred when a relatively high
rate of dose is likely to be needed over a long period, or for
acute conditions.

(b) *Trituration tablets*. Those substances which do not
lend themselves to potentizing by direct solution and
preparation according to the usual Hahnemannian potentizing process must be supplied in solid form in what are
termed trituration tablets. The usual strengths supplied are
3x and 6x available in the same size bottles as the medicated
tablets, 7g. and 25g. The trituration tablets are made from
trituration powder resulting from grinding the mother
substance with the required amount of pure lactose in the
prescribed manner. The dose is 2 tablets for adult, 1 for
child.

3   GRANULES
Of pure sugar. Often suitable for babies and very young
children. The dose is sufficient granules to cover the base of
a 7g. bottle cap direct on the tongue. Any medicine may
be put up in this form provided it is not a trituration. They
may also be put up in the form of individual doses of
approximately 750–1000mg. A 7g. vial of granules will
provide approximately 70 separate doses.

4   LIQUIDS
A potentized medicine may on occasion be required in a
liquid form either to be taken as a draught or in drop doses.
For a draught, one 7ml. vial of medicated 10% alcohol

solution is supplied; the whole of the contents to be taken direct from the vial.

For drop doses, dropper bottles of:

5ml. capacity, approximately	150	drops	(about	30	doses)
10ml.	,,	,,	320	,,	,,	64	,,
15ml.	,,	,,	475	,,	,,	95	,,
30ml.	,,	,,	960	,,	,,	192	,,
50ml.	,,	,,	1600	,,	,,	320	,,

are available. The potentized medicine is then dispensed in 20% alcohol and the dose is 3 to 5 drops in a little water at intervals as required by the prescriber.

Certain of the mother tinctures are also supplied in dropper bottles when required for internal medication.

A specimen prescription would be:

Crataegus φ 30ml. D.B.

m.x ex aq. n & m

or Chelidonium φ 30ml. D.B.

m.x ex aq. t.d.s.p.c.

5   GRANULED POWDERS

Individually wrapped 180mg. lactose powders containing a few granules are available. Packed in dozens they are useful when administering a few doses at the surgery or when visiting. It is only necessary to open the powder paper and sprinkle on a few granules from the medicated stock bottle in order to provide the doses.

Appendix 2

Nomenclature of Dilutions in Homoeopathic Pharmacy

The nomenclature used in homoeopathy has remained virtually unchanged from its introduction in the early part of the 19th century to the present day.

There are two methods of designating the degree of dilution present in the medication, that based on dilution in 10's and that based on dilution in 100's. The 10's scale is termed the decimal and the 100's scale, centesimal.

In the UK relatively few strengths are denoted as decimal, but the following will be seen:

$1x = 1/10 = 10^{-1}$

$3x = 1/1000 = 10^{-3}$

$6x = 1/1000000 = 10^{-6}$

The centesimal scale is much more frequently used, and the following numerals will be seen in the literature:

3 which is a dilution of $1/1000000 = 10^{-6}$

6   ,,   ,, ,,   ,,   ,, $1/1000000000000 = 10^{-12}$

12 which is a dilution of 10^{-24}

30 ,, ,, ,, ,, ,, 10^{-60}

200 ,, ,, ,, ,, ,, 10^{-400}

1000

or 1m ,, ,, ,, ,, ,, 10^{-2000}

The numbers are the conventional signs of homoeopathic medicine used to denote the strength or potency of preparation required. The strength denotes the degree of dilution of the solution used to moisten the solid forms of medicaments: tablets, pills or powder, etc.

The method of achieving the dilutions in the pharmacy is by use of individual containers which are filled to a predetermined capacity to provide a means of serial dilution, usually by 1 part in 100 parts in successive stages, thus it is necessary to utilize

6 vials to produce the 6c (10^{-12}) potency,

12 vials for the 12 (10^{-24})

30 vials for the 30 (10^{-60})

200 vials for the 200 (10^{-400})

and so on. At each separate stage of dilution the mixture is vigorously shaken, a process termed succussion.

It is apparent that the commonly used potencies of 6, 12, 30, 200 etc. do not contain any material quantity of the original solution in any preparation and it is evidently some intangible energy which is being produced and transferred to the solid dispensing forms. Consequently it is possible to produce tablets etc. by addition of drops of the required potency in redistilled ethanol. The number of drops need not be specific, sufficient to produce moistening of the whole contents of the vial in fact.

The various potencies may be used in a variety of circumstances, but in general low potencies:

3, 6 are used when there is clear pathological indication,

12, 30 may be more suited to functional disorder,

whilst 200, 1m are appropriate when the similimum is well

established or well defined symptoms of mood are present.

Despite the foregoing, the potencies may be used low for sensitive cases or chronic conditions, and high in acute states. It is very much a question of personal choice.

Rate of dosage;

Low and medium potency preparations may be given frequently, 2 tablets for an adult dose three or four times a day for a week, is not uncommon.

High potencies may be given less often, two or three times a day for 2 or 3 days, particularly in chronic conditions.

For acute conditions, high potencies may be given frequently until the patient responds.

Appendix 3

Common Cold Remedies

Aconite—Sudden chill from exposure to *cold dry winds*. Fever, thirst, roaring in ears. Sleeplessness. Sneezing, fluid clear hot water, with acutely inflamed throat, larynx sensitive to touch. Croup, dry short cough—distressing in children—loud dry spasmodic in anyone. Restless, anxious frightened. Sudden onset, worse at night.

ALLIUM CEPA—Cold with intense coryza, feels thick in head. Worse in warm room plus sneezing, eyes get red and there is profuse blandlachrymation, watering eyes and nose, acrid burning discharge from nose, and upper lip red and sore, better in open air.

ARSENICUM ALBUM—Pouring water from nose, excoriating upper lip. Some sneezing from irritation in one spot. Always catching cold from changes of weather. Begins in nose and travels to chest. Chilly, worse in draughts (*Hepar*), freezing, hugs fire (*Nux*). Chilly with burning, better from heat, restless, anxious, ice-cold blood through vessels. Asthmatic type of cough, dry hacking, no expectoration. Thirst for constant sips of cold water.

BELLADONNA—Sudden chill and violent onset of bronchitis.

Begins with sore red shiny throat. Intense mental excitement. Pain very acute, worse slightest movement, very violent pulsating headache. Flushed with intense burning heat, dilated pupils, very dry red tongue plus thirst.

BRYONIA—Cold going on to chest, hoarse and sore at back of throat. Goes on to cough which shakes him to bits and is very painful over top of chest. Holds chest on coughing, and head because of headache. Short racking dry cough, better lying affected side, much worse from motion. Very thirsty for long cold drinks—very hot—wants to be left alone—looks drugged and bluish. Follows *Gelsemium*. Very good for cough of measles.

GELSEMIUM—Colds which come on days after exposure in *warm, moist relaxing weather*. History of feeling chilled after being too hot some days before, and he does not at first notice windows open. Chilliness and shivers up and down back, in spite of being hot and sticky. Acute fluid coryza and sneezing. Looks heavy and bluish like early stage of a *Bryonia*, and often followed by *Bryonia*. Although hot, has cold extremities and is sitting by fire particularly in flu. Aching and heavy all over, with soreness in muscles. May get tickly cough or more croupy kind of cough. Headache severe in flu over head and eyes. Mild dislike of disturbance. Headache better, passing water. If excited will have sleepless night. *Thirstless* nearly always.

HEPAR SULPH.—Comes on in *cold dry weather*, often with sticking sensation like splinter in throat-paroxysms of dry teasing painful cough with very sore chest and throat, very hot but can't and won't move or be uncovered without feeling chilly. Sweats profusely but lies covered up to chin—no relief from sweat. Worse breathing cold air. Worse putting hand out of bed. Suffocative croupy cough. Very irritable and hypersensitive. Apt to quarrel with own shadow if nothing else about, particularly in flu and chest conditions.

General Remedies

ARNICA—For any injury or bruising, falls, fractures, before and after operation. Where there is history of old injury particularly if never well since, or if left with after-effects.

LACHESIS—Very hot remedy—bluish appearance left-sided remedy. All symptoms worse from heat, much worse from tight clothing or tight collar—must be loosened. Much worse after sleep, wakes feeling deadly. Better directly discharge starts in menstrual period. Great menopausal remedy, very loquacious and darts from subject to subject. Apt to be very jealous and suspicious.

NAT. MUR.—Patient of definite character and personality. Fairly well covered and tend to be broad. Tend to be scraggy in neck. Skin at rest always sallow. If excited come in flushed and look temporarily like *Phosph*. Flush fades and leaves them sallow and greasy looking. Coarse greasy hair. Crack in lower lip often. Herpes on lips with cold. Walks with rapid definite movements, meaning to get somewhere. Often sits down with hands shaking on putting down vegetables or parcels. Worse in hot room. Much worse from consolation. Resentful if they don't get attention, nasty if they do. *The greatest shock remedy*, hides feelings and avoids everyone. Often very fine people although apt to remember every slight since childhood. One of the greatest migraine and headache remedies. Wakes with headache, gets worse and worse until 11 or 12 noon then eases off as day gets cooler or lasts well into next night. Flashes and zig-zags before eyes with headache—headache worse using eyes. Sometimes sinking and empty, particularly at 11 a.m., may still feel sinking after meal. Salt craving, likes beer, fish and occasionally milk, but *may* have aversion to meat, coffee and fats.

NAT. SULPH.—Many of the same *Natrum* symptoms. Gets bronchitis in *warm wet weather*. Cough with dyspnoea. Has to sit up quickly to get rid of sputum or lie propped up—

greenish expectoration worse 4–5 a.m. Left-sided pneumonia.

PHOSPHORUS—Intelligent bright people with glint in the hair. Fine skin which flushes up quickly. Not damp skin but will sweat if nervous or from strenuous exercise. Full of apprehension if overtired. Thinks he is going to be ill, gets into state about business and what he has left undone. Fears and dreads marked. May fly into passion if opposed—very ashamed after—never nurses resentment like *Nat. mur.* Better sleep. Better rubbing. Fear dark, being alone, thunder, death, that something will happen. Unhappy in twilight—wants reassurance. Pneumonia remedy, lies on unaffected side, intensely thirsty, loves ice-cream, loves salt, loves cold water. Violent pain in chest on coughing, holds chest if tightness and pressure in chest. Better by pressure. One of chief *jaundice* remedies when it fits.

PULSATILLA—Gentle, yielding type. Weeps easily, better from sympathy. Wilts in heat, can't sit in sun. Apt to have late or delayed M.P. Often has wandering pains—rheumatism—often useful in single joint rheumatism. Hates fat of any kind. Rather likes sweets. Very little thirst. Cough worse evening, goes on and off until he expectorates.

RHUS TOX.—One of the greatest rheumatic and skin remedies. Lumbago worse before rain, much worse from cold, very bad on getting out of bed or chair. Better after movement, much better from warmth. All rheumatic complaints have same characteristics. Better from heat and movement, worse from cold, sitting or lying. Very thirsty. Very very restless. Can be used in pneumonias where these things fit. Very very good in shingles where patient walks about to ease pain, has constant hot applications or hot baths, checks 75%. Excellent in many skin complaints. Erysipelas after standing in cold wind. Patient very very restless, longs for heat, very thirsty, and in any skin trouble with restlessness, much worse from cold and much better from movement. Worse in bed because not moving—has to get up and walk about. Very thirsty.

SULPHUR—Untidy, hair won't lie down, dirty looking red faced, or greyish earthy appearance, shrivelled looking—'the lean dyspeptic' or 'the ragged philosopher' in appearance—redness of lips, eyelids, nostrils, anus—ravenous hunger, often worse 11 a.m., sometimes with emaciation. Marasmic baby with hot head and cold feet—puts everything into mouth. Craves fat of any kind. Children who help themselves to pats of butter. Likes sugar, salt, everything. Always tired, slow, lazy, selfish and hungry. Untidy and clumsy. Hates a bath. Worse from hot bath. Throws off bedclothes. Sticks feet out of bed. Slimy diarrhoea or looseness early a.m., or offensive and obstinate constipation, full of eruptions. Eczema, boils itching at night from warmth of bed. Worse from warm bath, warm room. Said to be very untidy but can appear very smart, but always something wrong—wrong socks, wears wrong suit, tie crooked, belt upside down. Burning indigestion, desire for cold drinks and ices, or eats a lot and drinks very little. Much worse from milk. Worse after sleep, eating, bathing. Slow growth and development. May fit patient in any illness, often finishes up a pneumonia, particularly after *Ars. alb.* Headaches, seven day periodicity, Sunday headache of workers. Long continued suppurations or ulcers. Old cases of gout. Very good for clearing ground and seeing patient clearly again.

Appendix 4

A brief description of the materials used in preparing the medicines supplied to doctors beginning in homoeopathy. These notes should be read in conjunction with Appendix 2 on nomenclature and the material on Homoeopathic Pharmacy. The 30th potency of each of the following is supplied in sugar granule form:

Aconite—Aconitum napellus

An alcoholic tincture of the fresh flowering plant is used to make the potencies.

Acidum phosphoricum—Phosphoric acid

A solution of the sticks of metaphosphoric acid is used to prepare the potencies.

Allium cepa—The mature onion

An alcoholic tincture of the fresh material is used in the preparation of the potencies.

Arnica montana

An alcoholic tincture of the fresh flowering plant is used to make the potencies.

Arsenicum album—White arsenic

A solution of arsenic is used to prepare the potencies.

Belladonna—Atropa belladonna

An alcoholic tincture of the fresh flowering plant is used to prepare the potencies.

Bryonia alba—White bryony

An alcoholic tincture of the fresh root is used to prepare the potencies.

Carbo vegetabilis—Charcoal from beech or birch

The crude substance is triturated with lactose and liquid potencies prepared from suitable strengths of triturate.

Gelsemium sempervirens—Yellow jasmine

An alcoholic tincture of the fresh root is used to prepare the potencies.

Hepar sulphuris—Impure calcium sulphide from fused oyster shells and sulphur

The crude substance is triturated with lactose and liquid potencies prepared from suitable strengths of triturate.

Kali bichromicum—Potassium bichromate

A solution of the substance is used to prepare the potencies.

Lycopodium clavatum—Club moss

The spores are triturated and an alcoholic tincture made from which the potencies are prepared.

Natrum muriaticum—Sodium chloride

The potencies are prepared from the dissolved salt.

Natrum sulphuricum—Sodium sulphate. Glauber's salt.

The potencies are prepared from a solution of the substance.

Nux vomica—Strychnos nux vomica

An alcoholic tincture is prepared from the seeds, from which the potencies are prepared.

Opium

The potencies are prepared from tincture of opium.

Phosphorus—White phosphorus

The potencies are prepared from an alcoholic solution of the substance.

Pulsatilla vulgaris—Pasque flower. Wind flower

An alcoholic tincture is made from the whole fresh flowering plant and potencies are prepared from this.

Sanguinaria canadensis—Blood root

An alcoholic tincture of the fresh rhizome is prepared and potencies are made from this.

Sepia officinalis—The fresh ink of the cuttlefish

The potencies are prepared from an alcoholic solution.

Silicea—Silicon oxide

Triturations of the fine powder are made and suitable strengths are used to make solutions from which the potencies are made.

Sulphur—Naturally occurring sulphur

Triturations of the crude substance are made, and a solution made at a suitable stage from which potencies are prepared.

Remedies,
their Abbreviations
and Common Names

Abies-c. *Abies canadensis* Canadian pitch fir

Abies-n. *Abies nigra* black spruce

Abrot. *Artemisia abrotanum* artemesia, lady's love

Absin. *Artemisia absinthium* common wormwood

Aca. *Acalypha indica* Indian acalypha

Acet-ac. *Aceticum acidum* Glacial acetic acid

Acon. *Aconitum napellus* monk's hood

Acon-c. *Aconitum cammarum* hybrid aconite

Acon-f. *Aconitum ferox* Himalayan wolf's bane

Act-sp. *Actea spicata* baneberry

Æsc. *Æsculus hippocastanum* horse chestnut

Æth. *Æthusa* fool's parsley

Agar. *Agaricus muscarius* fly agaric

Agar-em. *Agaricus emeticus* poison mushroom

Agar-ph. *Agaricus phalloides* death cap

Agn. *Agnus castus* vervain

Ail. *Ailanthus* tree of heaven

Alet. *Aletris farinosa* colic root, stargrass

All-c. *Allium cepa* red onion

All-s. *Allium sativum* garlic

Aloe *Aloe* aloe

Alumn. *Alumen* alum

Alum-m. *Aluminium metallicum* aluminium

Ambr. *Ambra* ambergris

Am-br. *Ammonium bromatum* bromide of ammonium

Am-c. *Ammonium carbonicum* sal volatile

Am-caust. *Ammonium causticum* spirits of hart's horn.

Ammc. *Ammoniacum* ammoniac plant juice

Am-m. *Ammonium muriaticum* sal ammoniac

Amph. *Amphisbæna* snake-lizard

Amyg. *Amygdalæ amaræ* aqua bitter almond

Amyl-n. *Amyl nitrosum* amyl nitrite

Anac. *Anacardium orientale* marking nut

Anag. *Anagallis arvensis* pimpernel

Anan. *Anantherum* anantherum

Ang. *Angustura* cusparia (from Angustura tree bark)

Anis. *Anisum stellatum* anise

Anth *Anthemis nobilis* chamomile

Anthr. *Anthracinum* anthrax

Ant-a. *Antimonium arsenitum* arsenate of antimony

Ant-c. *Antimonium crudum* sulphide of antimony

Ant-s. *Antimonium sulphuratum auratum* golden sulphuret of antimony

Aphis. *Aphis chenopodii glauci* aphis

Apis *Apis* honey-bee poison

Ap-g. *Apium graveolens* celery

Apoc. *Apocynum cannabinum* Indian hemp

Aral. *Aralia racemosa* spikenard

Aran. *Aranea diadema* papal cross spider

Arg-c. *Argentum cyanidum* silver cyanide

Arg-m. *Argentum metallicum* silver

Arg-n. *Argentum nitricum* silver nitrate

Arn. *Arnica montana* arnica, leopard's bane, fallkraut

Ars. *Arsenicum album* white oxide of arsenic

Ars-h. *Arsenicum hydrogenisatum* arseniuretted hydrogen

Ars-i. *Arsenicum iodatum* iodide of arsenic

Ars-m. *Arsenicum metallicum* metallic arsenic
Ars-s-f. *Arsenicum sulphuratum flavum* arsenious
    sulphide
Ars-s-r. *Arsenicum sulphuratum rubrum* arsenic
    disulphide
Art-v. *Artemesia vulgaris* mugwort
Arum-d. *Arum dracontium* green dragon
Arum-m. *Arum maculatum* lords and ladies,
    jack-in-the-pulpit
Arum-t. *Arum triphyllum* Indian turnip
Arund. *Arundo mauritanica* African reed
Asaf. *Ferula asafoetida* asafoetida (juice of the
    roots)
Asar. *Asarum* birthwort, wild ginger
Asc-c. *Asclepias cornuti (Syriaca)* silkweed
Asc-t. *Asclepias tuberosa* butterfly weed
Asim. *Asimina triloba* pawpaw
Aspar. *Asparagus* asparagus
Astac. *Astacus fluviatilis* European crawfish
Aster. *Asterias rubens* starfish
Atro. *Atropine* atropine
Aur. *Aurum metallicum* gold
Aur-m, *Aurum muriaticum* chloride of gold
Aur-m-n. *Aurum muriaticum natronatum* double
    chloride of gold and sodium
Aur-s. *Aurum sulphuratum* auric sulphide

Bad. *Badiaga* freshwater sponge
Bapt. *Baptisia tinctoria* wild indigo
Bart. *Bartfelder* acid spring
Bar-ac. *Baryta acetica* acetate of barium
Bar-c. *Baryta carbonica* carbonate of barium
Bar-m. *Baryta muriatica* chloride of barium
Bell. *Atropa belladonna* deadly nightshade
Bell-p. *Bellis perennis* daisy
Benz. *Benzenum* benzene
Benz-ac. *Benzoicum acidum* benzoic acid
Benz-n. *Benzenum nitricum* artificial oil of
    bitter almond
Berb. *Berberis vulgaris* barberry
Bism. *Bismuthum oxidum* bismuth
Blatta *Blatta orientalis* cockroach
Bol. *Boletus luricus* mushroom
Bor. *Borax* borax
Bor-ac. *Boracicum acidum* boric acid
Both. *Bothrops lanceolatus* yellow viper
Bov. *Bovista* puffball mushroom
Brach. *Brachyglottis* puka puka plant
Brom. *Bromium* bromine
Bruc. *Brucea antidysenterica* false angustura
Bry. *Bryonia alba* white bryony
Bufo, *Bufo* toad

Cact. *Cactus grandiflora* nightblooming cereus

Cadm. *Cadmium sulphuratum* sulphide of cadmium
Cahin. *Cahinca* cainca root
Caj. *Cajaputum*
Cal. *Caladium* caladium
Calc. *Calcarea carbonica* impure calcium
    carbonate
Calc-ac. *Calcarea acetica* impure calcium
    acetate
Calc-ar. *Calcarea arsenica* arsenite of lime
Calc-caust. *Calcarea causticum* quicklime
Calc-f. *Calcarea fluorica* calcium fluoride
Calc-i. *Calcarea iodata* iodide of lime
Calc-p. *Calcarea phosphorica* phosphate of lime
Calc-s. *Calcarea sulphurica* gypsum
Calc-sil. *Calcarea silicata* silicate of calcium
Calo. *Calotropis gigantea* tropical milkweed
Camph. *Cinnamomum camphora* camphor-tree
Cann-i. *Cannabis indica* hashish
Cann-s. *Cannabis sativa*
Canth. *Cantharis* blister beetle, Spanish fly
Caps. *Capsicum annuum* cayenne pepper
Carb-ac. *Carbolic acidumum* carbolic acid
Carb-an. *Carboneum animalis* animal carbon
Carb-h. *Carboneum hydrogenisatum* ethylene
Carb-o. *Carboneum oxygenisatum* carbon
    dioxide
Carb-s. *Carboneum sulphuratum* carbon
    bisulphide
Carb-v. *Carbo vegetabilis* vegetable carbon
Card-m. *Carduus marianus* thistle
Carl. *Carlsbad* Carlsbad water
Casc. *Cascarilla*
Cast. *Castoreum* oil of preputial gland of the
    beaver
Cast-eq. *Castor equi* castor of a horse's foreleg,
    rudimentary thumbnail of a horse
Cast-v. *Castanea vesca* chestnut
Caul. *Caulophyllum* papoose root, blue cohosh
Caust. *Causticum* causticum
Cean. *Ceanothus americanus* New Jersey tea
Cedr. *Simaba cedron* bitter damson
Cench. *Cenchris contortrix* copperhead snake
Cent. *Centaurea tagana* cornflower, sweet sultan
Cer-b. *Cereus bonplandii* nightblooming cereus
    (variety)
Cer-s. *Cereus serpentaria* nightblooming cereus
Chel. *Chelidonium majus* celandine
Chen-a. *Chenopodium anthelminticum* goosefoot,
    wormseed
Chen-v. *Chenopodium vulvaria* stinking
    goosefoot
Chim. *Chimaphila umbellata* prince's pine
Chin. *China Cinchona* quinine
Chin-a. *Chininum arsenicosum* arsenite of quinine
Chin-s. *Chininum sulphuricum* sulphate of quinine
Chion. *Chionanthus virginica* fringetree

Chlol. *Chloralum* chloral hydrate
Chlf. *Chloroform* chloroform
Chlor. *Chlorum* chlorine
Chr-ac. *Chromicum acidum* chromic acid
Cic. *Cicuta virosa* cowbane
Cimx. *Cimex* bedbug
Cimic. *Cimicifuga* crowfoot
Cina *Cina* seed of artemesia maritima
Cinch. *Cinchonium sulphuricum* quinine
Cinnb. *Cinnabaris* cinnabar
Cinn. *Cinnamomum* cinnamon
Cist. *Cistus* cistus canadensis
Cit-ac. *Citricum Acidum* citric acid
Cit-l. *Citrus limonum* lemon
Cit-v. *Citrus vulgaris* bitter orange
Clem. *Clematis* clematis
Cob. *Cobaltum* cobalt
Coca. *Erythroxylon coca* cocaine
Cocc. *Cocculus indicus* moonseed
Coc-c. *Coccus cacti* cochineal
Coch. *Cochlearia officinalis* scurvy grass
Cod. *Codeinum* codeine
Coff. *Coffea cruda* coffee berry
Coff-t. *Coffea tosta* roast coffee beans
Colch. *Colchicum autumnale* autumn crocus
Coll. *Collinsonia* horse balm
Coloc. *Citrullus colocynthis* bitter apple
Com. *Comocladia* guao
Con. *Conium maculatum* poison hemlock
Cond. *Condurango* condor vine
Conv. *Convallaria majalis* lily-of-the-valley
Cop. *Copaiva* balsam of copaiva
Cor-r. *Corallium rubrum* red coral
Cori-r. *Coriaria ruscifolia* coriaria
Corn. *Cornus circinata* dogberry
Corn-f. *Cornus florida* American dogwood
Corn-s. *Cornus sericea* squawberry, dwarf cornel
Croc. *Crocus* crocus
Crot-c. *Crotalus cascavella* Brazilian rattlesnake
Crot-h. *Crotalus horridus* rattlesnake
Crot-t. *Croton tiglium* croton oil
Cub. *Cubeba* pepper
Culx. *Culex moscæ* mosquito
Cupr. *Cuprum* copper
Cupr-ar. *Cuprum arsenicosum* arsenite of copper
Cupr-s. *Cuprum sulphuricum* sulphate of copper
Cur. *Curare* curare
Cycl. *Cyclamen* sow bread, cyclamen
Cypr. *Cypripedium* wild orchid, lady slipper, mocassin flower

Daph. *Daphne indica* daphne, spurge laurel
Der. *Derris pinnata* insecticide (from the bean)
Dig. *Digitalis purpurea* foxglove

Dios. *Dioscorea* yam
Dirc. *Dirca palustris* leatherwood, moosewood
Dol. *Dolichos pruriens* mucuna
Dor. *Doryphora* Colorado potato-bug
Dros. *Drosera* sundew
Dulc. *Solanum dulcamara* bittersweet

Echi. *Echinacea angustifolia* cone-flower
Elaps. *Elaps corallinus* coral-snake
Elat. *Elaterium* squirting cucumber
Epig. *Epigea repens* trailing arbutus
Equis. *Equisetum* horsetail
Erig. *Erigeron, Leptilon canadense* fleabane
Ery-a. *Eryngium aquaticum* buttonsnake root
Eucal. *Eucalyptus globulus* gumtree
Eug. *Eugenia jambos* rose apple
Euon. *Euonymus europæus* spindletree
Eup-per. *Eupatorium perfoliatum* boneset, thoroughwort
Euph. *Euphorbium* euphorbia gum
Euphr. *Euphrasia* eyebright
Eupi. *Eupion* woodtar

Fago. *Fagopyrum* buckwheat
Ferr. *Ferrum* iron
Ferr-ar. *Ferrum arsenicosum* arsenate of iron
Ferr-i. *Ferrum iodatum* iodide of iron
Ferr-m. *Ferrum muriaticum* ferrous chloride
Ferr-ma. *Ferrum magneticum* lodestone
Ferr-p. *Ferrum phosphoricum* phosphate of iron
Ferr-pic. *Ferrum picricum* picrate of iron
Ferr-s. *Ferrum sulphuricum* sulphate of iron
Fl-ac. *Fluoricum acidum* hydrofluoric acid
Form. *Formica* formic acid (from ants)

Gamb. *Gambogia* gamboge, gummigutti
Gels. *Gelsemium* jasmine
Genist. *Genista* broom
Gent-c. *Gentian cruciata* cross-leaved gentian
Gent-l. *Gentian lutea* yellow gentian, felwort
Ger. *Geranium maculatum* crane's bill
Gins. *Ginseng Panax schinseng* ginseng root
Glon. *Glonoin* nitroglycerine
Gnaph. *Gnaphalium* cudweed, old balsam
Goss. *Gossypium* cotton
Gran. *Granatum* extract of pomegranate bark
Graph. *Graphites* plumbago, black lead
Grat. *Gratiola* hedge hyssop
Grin. *Grindelia robusta* gum plant
Guaj. *Guaiacum* lignum vitæ
Guar. *Paullinia corbilis* guarana, Brazilian cocoa
Guare. *Guarea* ballweed
Gymn. *Gymnocladus* Kentucky coffee tree

Hæm. *Hæmotoxylon campechianum* logwood
Ham. *Hamamelis* American witch hazel
Hecla. *Hecla lava* volcanic ash
Hell. *Helleborus niger* christmas rose
Helo. *Heloderma* gila monster
Helon. *Helonias* unicorn root devil's bit
Hep. *Hepar sulphuris calcareum* calcium sulphide
Hipp. *Hippomanes* meconium deposit
Hippoz. *Hippozaenium* farcine
Ho. *Homarus* lobster
Hura *Hura braziliensis* sap of the sandbox tree
Hydr. *Hydrastis canadensis* golden seal
Hydrang. *Hydrangea* hydrangea
Hydr-ac. *Hydrocyanic acidum* prussic acid
Hydrc. *Hydrocotyle* Indian pennywort
Hyos. *Hyosyamus niger* henbane
Hyper. *Hypericum perforatum* St John's wort

Iber. *Iberis* bitter candytuft
Ign. *Strychnos ignatia* St Ignatius bean
Ill. *Illicium anisatum* anise
Indg. *Indigo* indigo
Inul. *Inula* elecampane, scabwort
Iod. *Iodum* iodine
Ip. *Ipecacuanha* ipecacuanha
Ir-fl. *Iris florentina* orris root, white flag
Ir-fœ. *Iris foetidissima* stinking iris
Iris. *Iris versicolor* iris, blue flag

Jab. *Pilocarpus jaborandi* jaborandi (dried leaflets of)
Jac. *Jacaranda caroba* caroba
Jal. *Jalapa* jalap
Jatr. *Jatropha* purging nut
Jug-c. *Juglans cinerea* butternut
Jug-re. *Juglans regia* English walnut
Juni. *Juniperus virginia* red cedar

Kali-ar. *Kali arsenicosum* potassium arsenite Fowler's solution
Kali-bi. *Kali bichromicum* bichromate of potash
Kali-br. *Kali bromatum* bromide of potash
Kali-c. *Kali carbonicum* potassium carbonate
Kali-ch. *Kali chloricum* potassium chlorate
Kali-cy. *Kali cyanatum* potassium cyanide
Kali-fer. *Kali ferrocyanatetum* yellow prussiate of potash
Kali-io. *Kali iodatum* potassium iodide
Kali-ma. *Kali manganicum* permanganate
Kali-n. *Kali nitricum* saltpetre of potash

Kali-p. *Kali phosphoricum* phosphate of potassium
Kali-s. *Kali sulphuricum* potassium sulphate
Kalm. *Kalmia* American laurel
Kao. *Kaolin* china clay
Kiss. *Kissengen* Kissengen water
Kreos. *Kreosote* creosote

Lac-c. *Lac caninum* bitch's milk
Lac-d. *Lac defloratum* skimmed milk
Lac-f. *Lac felinum* cat's milk
Lach. *Lachesis* bushmaster (poison of)
Lachn. *Lanchnanthes* red root spirit weed
Lac-ac. *Lacticum acidum* lactic acid
Lact. *Lactuca* lettuce
Lam. *Lamium* white nettle
Lap-a. *Lapis albus* silico fluoride of calcium
Lath. *Lathyrus* chick-pea
Lat-m. *Latrodectus mactans* black widow spider
Laur. *Laurocerasus* cherry laurel
Leci. *Lecithin* (constituent of egg yolk)
Led. *Ledum* Labrador tea
Lem-m. *Lemna minor* duckweed
Lep. *Lepidium bonariense* peppergrass, Brazilian cress
Lept. *Leptandra virginica* tall speedwell
Lil-t. *Lilium tigrinum* tiger lily
Lith-c. *Lithium carbonicum*
Lith-m. *Lithium muriaticum*
Lob-c *Lobelia cardinalis* red lobelia
Lob-i. *Lobelia inflata* Indian tobacco
Lob-sy. *Lobelia syphilitica* blue lobelia
Lyco. *Lycopodium* club moss
Lycopers. *Lycopersicum* tomato
Lycopus *Lycopus virginicus* bugle-weed
Lyss. *(Lyssin) Hydrophobinum* saliva of a rabid dog

Mag-c. *Magnesia carbonica* magnesium carbonate
Mag-m. *Magnesia muriatica* magnesium chloride
Mag-ph. *Magnesia phosphorica* phosphate of magnesia
Mag-s. *Magnesia sulphurica* Epsom salts
Mag-arc. *Magnetis polis arcticus* North pole of a magnet
Mag-aust. *Magnetis polis australis* South pole of a magnet
Maland. *Malandrinum* sallenders (scale disease of the hind leg of a horse)
Man. *Mancinella* manchineel juice
Mang. *Manganum* manganese
Mang-m. *Manganum muriaticum* chloride of manganese

Med. *Medorrhinum* leucorrhoea, gonorrhoea virus
Meli. *Melilotus* sweet clover
Meny. *Menyanthes* buckwheat
Meph. *Mephitis* skunk scent
Merc. *Mercurius* mercury
Merc-c. *Mercurius corrosivus* mercuric chloride
Merc-cy. *Mercurius cyanatus* mercuric cyanide
Merc-d. *Mercurius dulcis* calomel
Merc-i-f. *Mercurius iodatus flavus* proto-iodide of mercury
Merc-n. *Mercurius nitrosus* nitrate of mercury
Merc-sul. *Mercurius sulphuricus* yellow sulphate of mercury
Merl. *Mercurialis perennis* dog's mercury
Mez. *Mezereum* dried bark of daphne, spurge olive
Mill. *Achillea millefolium* yarrow
Mit. *Mitchella* partridgeberry
Mosch. *Moschus* musk
Murx. *Murex* purple dye
Mur-a. *Muriaticum acidum* hydrochloric acid
Mygal. *Mygale lasiodora* tropical woolly spider
Myric. *Myrica cerifera* wax myrtle, bayberry
Myris. *Myristica sebifera* Brazilian ucuba

Naja *Naja* hooded cobra
Narcot. *Narcotinum* alkaloid of opium
Nat-a. *Natrum arsenicatum* sodium arsenate
Nat-c. *Natrum carbonicum* sodium carbonate
Nat-h. *Natrum hypophosphorosum* sodium hypophosphite
Nat-m. *Natrum muriaticum* sodium chloride salt
Nat-n. *Natrum nitricum* nitrate of soda
Nat-p. *Natrum phosphoricum* phosphate of soda
Nat-s. *Natrum sulphuricum* sodium sulphate
Nicc. *Niccolum* nickel
Nit-ac. *Nitricum acidum* nitric acid
Nit-m-ac. *Nitricum muriaticum acidum* aqua regia
Nit-s-d. *Nitri spiritus dulcis* sweet spirits of nitre
Nuph. *Nuphar luteum* yellow pond lily
Nux-m. *Nux moschata* nutmeg
Nux-v. *Nux vomica* strychnine, poison nut

Oci. *Ocimum canum* Brazilian alfavaca
Œna. *Œnanthe crocata* hemlock dropwort
Olnd. *Oleander* rose laurel
Ol-an. *Oleum animale* animal oil
Ol-j. *Oleum jecoris aselli* cod liver oil
Onos. *Onosmodium* false gromwell
Op. *Opium* opium
Orig. *Origanum marjorana* marjoram
Osmium *Osmium*

Pæon. *Pæonia* peony

Pall. *Palladium*
Pareir. *Pareira brava* virgin vine
Par. *Paris quadrifolia* herb-Paris, true love
Pen. *Penthorum* Virginia stonecrop
Peti *Petiveria* guinea-hen weed
Petr. *Petroleum*
Fetros. *Petroselinum* parsley
Phal. *Phallus impudicus* stinkhorn
Phasc. *Phaseolus nanus* dwarf bean
Phel. *Phellandrium* water dropwort
Phos. *Phosphorus*
Ph-ac. *Phosphoricum acidum* phosphoric acid
Phys. *Physostigma* calabar bean
Phyt. *Phytolacca* pokeweed
Pic-ac. *Picricum acidum* picric acid
Pin-s. *Pinus silvestris* Scots pine
Pip-m. *Piper methysticum* kavakava juice
Pip-n. *Piper nigrum* black peppercorn
Plan. *Plantago* ribwort, plantain
Plat. *Platinum*
Plect. *Plectranthus* spur-flower
Plb. *Plumbum* lead
Plumbg. *Plumbago littoralis* plumbago
Podo *Podophyllum* may-apple
Polyg. *Polygonum hydropiperoides* smart weed
Pop. *Populus canadensis* balm of gilead
Poth. *Pothos foetidus* skunk cabbage
Prun. *Prunus spinosa* sloe
Psor. *Psorinum* itch
Ptel. *Ptela trifoliata* hop tree, water ash
Pulx. *Pulex irritans* flea
Puls. *Pulsatilla vulgaris* wind flower
Pul-n. *Pulsatilla nuttaliana* American pasque-flower
Pyrog. *Pyrogenium* artificial sepsin
Pyrus *Pyrus americana* American mountain ash

Rad. *Radium bromide*
Ran-b. *Ranunculus bulbosus* buttercup
Ran-s. *Ranunculus sceleratus* crow foot, marsh buttercup
Raph. *Raphanus* radish
Rat. *Ratanhia* ratany root
Rheum *Rheum* rhubarb
Rhod. *Rhododendron* rhododendron
Rhus-a. *Rhus aromatica* fragrant sumac
Rhus-t. *Rhus toxicodendron* poison ivy
Rhus-v. *Rhus venenata* poison sumac
Rob. *Robinia* locust tree, false acacia
Rumx. *Rumex crispus* curled dock
Ruta *Ruta* rue

Sabad. *Sabadilla* sabadilla (cevadilla) seed
Sabal. *Sabal serrulata* Florida palm, saw palmetto

Sabin. *Juniperis sabina* juniper savin
Sal-ac. *Salicylicum acidum* aspirin
Sal-n. *Salix nigricans* black willow
Samb. *Sambucus nigra* elder
Sang. *Sanguinaria* blood root
Sanic. *Sanicula aqua* Sanicula spring water
Sarr. *Sarracenia* cobra plant, pitcher plant
Sars. *Sarsaparilla* sarsparilla
Scut. *Scutellaria* skull cap
Sec. *Secale cornum* ergot of rye
Sel. *Selenium*
Senec. *Senecio aureus* golden ragwort
Seneg. *Polygala senega* seneca, snake root
Sep. *Sepia* cuttlefish ink
Sil. *Silicea* silica, flint
Sin-a. *Sinapis alba* white mustard
Sin-n. *Sinapis nigra* black mustard
Sol-m. *Solanum mammosum*
Sol-n. *Solanum nigrum* black night shade
Sol-o. *Solanum oleraceum* juquerioba
Sol-t-ae. *Solanum tuberosum aegrotans* diseased
    potato
Spig. *Spigelia* pink root
Spig-m. *Spigelia marilandica* worm grass
Spira. *Spiranthes (Gyrostachys)* wild ground
    orchid, lady's tresses
Spong. *Spongia* sponge
Squil. *Squilla maritima* sea onion
Stach. *Stachys betonica* hedge nettle, wood
    betony
Stann. *Stannum* tin
Staph. *Delphinium staphisagria* stavesacre
Stel. *Stellaria media* chickweed
Stict. *Sticta pulmonaria* lichen, lungwort
Still. *Stillingia sylvatica* queen's delight,
    queen's root
Stram. *Stramonium* thorn apple
Stront. *Strontium*
Stry. *Strychninum* alkaloid of *nux vomica*
Sulph. *Sulphur*
Sul-ac. *Sulphuricum acidum* sulphuric acid
Sul-i. *Sulphur iodatum* iodide of sulphur
Sumb. *Sumbul* musk root
Syph. *Syphilinum* lueticum, syphilitic virus

Tab. *Tabacum* tobacco
Tanac. *Tanacetum* tansy
Tann. *Tannin* tannic acid (from the leaves
    and bark of tea)
Tarax. *Taraxacum* dandelion
Tarent. *Tarentula* tarantula
Tarent-c. *Tarentula cubensis* Cuban tarantula
Tax. *Taxus baccata* European yew

Tell. *Tellurium*
Tep. *Teplitz* Teplitz spring water
Ter. *Terebinthina* turpentine
Teucr. *Teucrium marum verum* cat thyme
Thal. *Thallium*
Thea *Thea* tea
Ther. *Theridion* orange spider
Thuj. *Thuja* arbor vitae
Til. *Tilia* linden, lime tree
Trif-p. *Trifolium pratense* red clover
Tril. *Trillium pendulum* trillium
Trom. *Trombidium muscae domesticae* house fly
    mites
Tub. *Tuberculinum* tuberculous sputum
Tus-f. *Tussilage farfara* coltsfoot

Upa. *Upas* upas tree
Uran. *Uranium nitricum* nitrate of uranium
Urt-u. *Urtica urens* stinging nettle
Ust. *Ustilago* corn smut
Uva. *Uva ursi* bearberry

Vac. *Vaccininum*
Valer. *Valeriana* valerian
Vario. *Variolinum* small pox
Verat. *Veratrum album* white hellebore
Verat-v. *Veratrum viride* white American
    hellebore
Verb. *Verbascum* mullein
Vesp. *Vespa* wasp
Vib. *Viburnum opulus* high cranberry
Vinc. *Vinca* periwinkle, myrtle
Viol-o. *Viola odorata* violet
Viol-t. *Viola tricolor* pansy, hearts ease
Vip. *Vipera* viper
Visc. *Viscum album* European mistletoe

Wye. *Wyethia* poison weed

Xan. *Xanthoxylum* prickly ash, tooth-ache tree

Yuc. *Yucca* yucca

Zinc. *Zincum* zinc
Zinc-m. *Zincum muriaticum* chloride of zinc
Zinc-s. *Zincum sulphuricum* sulphate of zinc
    white vitrinole
Zing. *Zingiber* ginger
Ziz. *Zizia* meadow parsnip, wild rice

Index